"Never give up", Recovery is a Life Sentence:

A Guide to Dignified Stroke Recovery

By John Grant
(Five Year Recovery Edition)

Dedicated to:

Gen, the most important person in the world. A better wife and companion, no one could ever ask for:

She inspires me to transcend the mediocrities of life, and transcend them I will.
In quite moments, she thrills my heart and fills my soul, with joy and gratitude
When I ponder life's purposes, and look for answers eagerly,
She comes to me in my heart of hearts and tells me she belongs there.
Love compels me to discover unto her my hidden self, and make her mine forever, and make her mine I will.
-John Grant, c. 1993

Special Thanks to:

My good friend Terrance P. Howard for editing assistance and other insights.

An imprint of Kindle Direct publishing
Seattle, Washington, 98101 U.S.A.
Text copyright © 2018 by John Grant
All rights reserved, including the right of reproduction in whole or in part in any form.
Manufactured in the United States of America
For Kindle Direct Publishing 2020
20 21 22
The Library of Congress has catalogued the first edition, as follows:
John Grant, 2019-
Never Give Up!: Recovery is a Life Sentence / John Grant
p. cm.
Summary: A guide to dignified stroke recovery.
ISBN-9 71795732604
ISBN-9 798555872883

## Table of Contents

Introduction .................................................... 9

Part I: Why? [Denial] ............................ 24

    Chapter One: You are you (How did this happen to you?) ................... 25

    Chapter Two: Why not you? ............. 29

    Chapter Three: Never Again! ............ 34

    Chapter Four: Keep It in Perspective ................................................. 40

Part II: Be Grateful [Coping with Anger] .......... 46

    Chapter five: Seriously? (Did this really just happen to me?) ................. 47

    Chapter Six: Depression ..................... 53

    Chapter Seven: Therapy .................... 63

    Chapter eight: What You Don't Know ................................................. 69

    Chapter nine: I'm done (This is the end of my rope) ................................. 76

    Chapter ten: Win the Race ................ 86

Part III: Work Your Butt Off [There is no Negotiating Here] ............................. 94

    Chapter eleven: Start Every Day with a Plan ....................................... 95

Chapter Twelve: Gettin'er Done! (You've got this.)....................................99

Chapter Thirteen: It's No Picnic (Recovery is work)..............................105

Chapter Fourteen: "When Will It Ever End?" I'm sorry that sounded an awful lot like a complaint. ..........112

Part IV: Something For Everyone [Advice For Others in Your Life]........117

Chapter Fifteen: Stroke Widow......118

Chapter Sixteen: The Well Intentioned Spouse ............................131

Chapter Seventeen: Stroke from your young child's perspective........139

Chapter Eighteen: A script for explaining stroke to small children.....................................................146

Part V: Reach Out [Here's Where You Can Negotiate] .........................................150

Chapter Nineteen: Take a Chance 151

Chapter Twenty: Friends and Family (you're most immediate source of help).....................155

Chapter Twenty-One: Church and Community ............................................159

Chapter Twenty-Two: Be ready when help is offered .......... 164

Part VI: Coping with loss [Acceptance] .......... 170

Chapter Twenty-Three: Career ...... 171

Chapter Twenty-Four: Yourself ...... 178

Chapter Twenty-Five: Friends and Family .......... 183

Part VII: Be Inspirational [Getting Past the Grief] .......... 190

Chapter Twenty-Six: Without Even Trying (You are an inspiration) ...... 191

Chapter Twenty-Seven: Just a Little Bit More (A little extra makes all the difference) .......... 195

Chapter Twenty-Eight: But I'm Tired .......... 200

Part VIII: More with Less [Rebuilding Your Life] .......... 205

Chapter Twenty-Nine: Embrace Life .......... 206

Chapter Thirty: Deny Discouragement .......... 211

Chapter Thirty-One: Silver Linings .......... 215

Chapter Thirty-Two: Surround Yourself (You can never have enough friends)..................220

Chapter Thirty-Three: Freak of Nature......................................224

## Other Books by John Grant

### Once Upon a Time: A guide to bedtime storytelling
(Non-fiction)
Available on Amazon.com     eBook | Paperback

### Selected: The Oracle Chronicles (Fiction)
Available on Amazon.com     eBook | Paperback

### The White Tower Series, the Boghy man trilogy
(Fiction)
Available on Amazon.com
Book One: Gone but not forgotten   eBook | Paperback
Book Two: The Boghyman strikes again eBook | Paperback
Book Three: Too close to home   eBook | Paperback

**Introduction**

What is this about stroke recovery being a life sentence? I know, you were told it was temporary and that is partially true. I know that "life sentence" sounds harsh, but better that you know now. You will spend years regaining what you lost during the stroke, and then you'll spend the rest of your life maintaining what you've regained. If you are reading this then you have likely suffered a stroke, or you know someone who has, and as bad as it may feel or look now, it is not the end of the world. However, life will never seem the same again. That should not discourage you, though when you think about it, when has life ever been the same. It changes constantly, from minute to minute and from day to day. Likely, your life was exactly the way you created it to be. It was probably not perfect, but I imagine you were comfortable in it. As a result of the stroke, this is now the beginning of a new chapter in your life, or even a new book. The severity of your stroke will determine which it is. The phrase "different strokes for different folks," is completely accurate. Your stroke and the extent it has affected, and will continue to affect your life, is entirely unique to you. That is not to say that no one knows what you are going through. The mechanics of everyone's brain are basically the same. You're not alone...you're so not alone. I am here and I want to help, and there are others around you who feel the same way.

    Let's be absolutely clear on this point. It is not undignified to ask for—or accept—help from others. Stroke recovery is a long term process, and you should accept help whenever possible. It is, in fact, pitiful to watch someone fail over and over again when they could succeed if they would only accept a little help. I wrote this book to help you see the road ahead, and some of the common pitfalls you will likely face, and the resources available to you on your journey. None of what I have to tell you is new, but it may be new to you, what I have to offer is recovery from my perspective. My personal goal is to have a complete and total recovery, with no discernable residual stroke effect. Your journey of recovery, on the other hand, will be as unique as you and your stroke are.

As you begin this journey, you may be tempted to express your frustration. You have legitimate and justifiable gripes, but I encourage you to limit your self-expressions to a more positive approach. It is more dignified to be optimistic, especially under serious consequences. This is not about making other people happy and more comfortable with you. Screw that. This is about regaining and maintaining your dignity. Your two primary goals are, to recover your functionality, and to regain your dignity in the process. I wrote this book to help you do both, from the perspective of my own recovery experience and what has worked for me and others I know.

Now, let's get scientific for a moment. Throughout your life, your brain has developed neuropathways—habits—that your brain facilitates without any conscious help from you. Subconsciously, or without any effort on your part, your brain translates your habitual choices into autonomic actions. That is why you suddenly realize that you took a bite of that donut, despite your conscious choice to cut carbs out of your diet. Through habitual choices, you have taught, or conditioned, your brain to do things for you without having to focus; like always eating a donut when one is available. The sight and smell of the donut trigger your autonomic system and you pick up the donut and take a bite. In the same way, if you want your brain to ignore the donut, you have to train it to do so.

There are certain habits that you had stored in the stroke affected part of your brain that are now no longer accessible. Like bad sectors of a computer hard drive, your brain can no longer access the information that had been stored there. It's not that something is interfering with your brain's ability to access the information, like a computer virus distracts and confuses the operating system of a computer. It is more like the information is simply gone. To continue our computer analogy, if you delete a file from the hard drive of your computer you can always go to the trash to restore it, but if you empty the trash, then except for some expensive restoration software the file is gone. There's no recovery program for retrieving brain files lost due to stroke. You're starting all over from scratch, in some respects, and "scratch" in the case of stroke recovery means infancy. I know it hurts to hear that, but there it is, so deal with it.

As I understand it, and have witnessed for myself by watching my own children, as babies, you first learned to roll from side to side, then quite by accident, you roll over. You then learned to scoot yourself along the floor by moving your arms and legs, and eventually, you trained your brain to contort your body into a hands and knees "kneeling position" and you started to crawl. In every phase of this process, you tried and failed and tried again until you figured it out. It was not frustrating, because it was all new and you had no basis for judging your progress. At first, you had no idea what to expect. Gradually you began to realize what would happen as you moved your body in certain patterns. Nothing had been taken away from you, everything was new and exciting. Ultimately you began to develop expectations of what would happen when you made certain choices, and when your expectations were not met, you complained in a loud and annoying way. Complaining is not always expressed in words. Any expression of dissatisfaction will be interpreted by others as a complaint. Complaining in your case is justifiable, but it is certainly not dignified, and it sends the wrong message to your brain.

As a stroke survivor, you are or will be experiencing the stages of grief and loss, so right now complaining may be all you want to do, perhaps not as loud and annoying as an infant, but since the stroke, your expectations are not being met and so you may want to complain. However, complaining is only going to make you look childish and rob you of all of the personal dignity you have been working so hard to re-acquire. I have observed that most human beings want others to respect and admire them. One common opposite of respect is pity, and anyone who craves that has a distorted view of life. Pity, I have learned, cannot exist in the same state as respect and admiration or even dignity. So, I have found that if someone pities me, they cannot admire me for the same reason and in the same moment. Like most human beings I probably don't want to be pitied. Perhaps you are the same. However, you have suddenly found yourself in what you might consider a pitiful state. Despite your hard earned and well deserved pre-stroke personal dignity, you are now someone that others may naturally want to pity. Don't let that discourage you. Everyone knows you didn't consciously chose this outcome for yourself. If you are like the typical stroke survivor, you just want everything to go back to the way it was before the stroke. You're pre-stroke life may seem like a dream now. Before the stroke, you interacted with the world the way everyone else in your circle of the universe did; however, you may now feel like a freak-show anytime you attempt the simplest and most mundane tasks.

Your friends and family do not have to vocalize it, you can see the pity building in their eyes. You're not how you used to be, you know it, and they can see it. You no longer move the way others have become accustomed to seeing you move and they may want to respond with pity. Pity, in and of itself, is not a bad thing. It is an expression of empathy, which we should all foster in ourselves. That you do not want to be pitied is another subject all together. It would not be inappropriate for you to say that you appreciate the emotional support of others, but you would rather not be pitied, because you do not see yourself as pitiful. You are doing the best you can to retrain your brain to do things you have not had to teach it since you were an infant. Only those suffering from a brain injury, or the loss of a limb ever have to retrain their brain in the intense way you are now experiencing. What's worse, you are attempting to reverse engineer the whole process, because you already know what you expect. I encourage you to keep in mind that as a child you learned everything gradually. One movement built on another until you had total control of your body. As an adult, you already know what you can or could expect from your body and you're attempting to recreate something you've lost. In this case, it is your expectations that are creating your biggest hurdles. If you had no idea what to expect, you wouldn't get so frustrated or feel so awkward. This process would seem normal.

As a baby, you were the recipient of as much pity as you may be getting now, if not more. As a baby, every time you tried to stand up and toppled over, you were responded to with pity, but you interpreted it as love and caring. Pity at that time of your life was a good thing. Someone would rush over and pick you up, give you a little cuddle and a kiss and praise you for trying so hard. It was okay then because it supported your self-image. You were a toddler, and for all you knew, that's how people were supposed to treat you. However, your self-image has evolved over time and now you think that pity is no longer an acceptable way for people to treat you. Your personal definition of dignity rails against the concept of being treated like a toddler. Your expectations aren't being met, so you may be likely to complain. However, remember that complaining is not dignified.

It has been said that there are five stages of grief (Denial, Anger, Bargaining, Depression and Acceptance). You may not experience them in that order and you may not experience every stage. In fact, from my own experience, I've learned that you can fast forward through the first three and get stuck in depression. I have discovered through painful experience that to maintain your dignity throughout this grieving and recovery process you just have to let go of dignity as you have come to define it. I don't mean that you should intentionally behave in an undignified manner. What I'm saying is stop worrying about whether people respect and admire you and stop complaining about being treated like a child. I promise you that if you submit willingly to the notion that you are starting from scratch, then people will respect and admire you as they see you work hard at recovering. I promise you that this approach will help your dignity to remain intact.

Dignity in the eyes of others is earned. You've probably spent a lifetime earning it, but that lifetime is either over, or dramatically altered. You're laying a new foundation, except people who know you from before are more likely to give you the benefit of the doubt. Earning respect and admiration should not be as hard to achieve this time, but it does require effort and dedication on your part. I appreciate and sympathize with the strain you're under. I have been there and I know how unfair it seems. Here's another analogy that might open your eyes to this concept. Remember when you were a teenager, struggling to exert your independence, and wanting to be treated like an adult? You may experience stroke recovery in a very similar way, and like being a teenager, it will take time and consistent effort on your part to achieve the ultimate outcome you desire. My own recovery is still in progress, so you and I are on this journey together. I know that you can do this. Thank you, because, your struggle inspires me, and I hope that mine will inspire you too.

# Part I: Why? [Denial]

## *Chapter One: You are you (How did this happen to you?)*

At first, you probably didn't want to believe that this was happening to you; however, a stroke leaves very little room for doubt. Once you accepted what has happened, the first question you probably asked yourself, is "Why me?" It's a reasonable question, but one without an answer. Healthcare professionals can do a fair job of telling you "what a stroke is", but the answer as to why you had a stroke, that is all mixed up in a combination of genetics, diet and environment. The reason for your stroke is as individual as you. If you spent enough time and money you could probably pin point the exact contributing factors to your stroke, but knowing won't bring back your missing brain cells. The most you can hope for is to know how to prevent it from happening in the future and for that there is an answer. However, you're not going to like the answer when you get it. Stroke lesson number one, don't ask questions you don't want the answer too.

If you're asking "why" anyway, you're on a wild-goose chase, or worse, like a dog (a severely disabled dog), you're chasing your own tail. Focus your attention on overcoming the effects of the stroke and preventing more strokes in the future. I have found that being proactive rather than reactive will carry you much farther in this process.

Dignity, as I understand it, demands that you accept the inevitable dead-end of certain questions and move on with life. If you get stuck in an endless loop and become fixated on anything that leads nowhere, not only will you lose respect and admiration, but your entire mental stability may come into question.

Actionable Recovery Strategies:
1. *Why me*, is a question without an answer. Focus on questions you can answer.
2. Even if someone could answer the question, the answer won't give you back your lost brain cells. Stop chasing ghosts and look for answers that will inspire you to focus more on your recovery.
3. Recovery from this stroke, and prevention of future strokes should be the primary focus of your search for answers. Look for the answers to the question, "What can I do?"

4. You probably wouldn't like the answer to the question "why" anyway. There are so many more productive and effective questions you should be asking.
5. You can protect the dignity you have already regained by not becoming fixated on dead-end questions.

## *Chapter Two: Why not you?*

Ask yourself, "What choices have I made in my life to prevent stroke." If you're like most of the human race, the answer is nothing. To a great extent you were asking for the stroke. The question now is what choices are you going to make from now on to avoid a future stroke? You should be receiving extensive therapy to recover the functionality of your body and brain. Along with this therapy you have been given simple repetitive exercises to practice at home. Yes, I'm going to say it, do your home therapies! You may not remember how you learned as a baby. But, if you're normal you persistently practiced certain movements over and over again in a single minded determination to gain control of your body. In order to regain control of your body, you need the same single-minded determination. Don't let your infant self, show you up. Be that dedicated person who everyone can admire and respect. You can no longer afford to sit around and neglect your body; assuming that it will always be there for you. Life has forced you to look in the mirror and see the truth, this now is your life and your responsibility.

It's been estimated that every year 600,000 people in the United States alone will suffer their first stroke and another 200,000 will suffer another stroke. So at current population rates, approximately 2% of the U.S. population suffer their first stroke every year. I suppose that means that inside of thirty years most of us will be recovering from a stroke. As it happens, the vast number of stroke sufferers are over 65 years old, but that particular statistic did me no good when I suffered a stroke at the age of 51. Hard as it may be to accept, you're a statistic now, but you might as well get used to it. Stroke, it turns out, is the leading cause of long-term disability in the U.S. That's "long-term" not permanent disability. I want you to take comfort in knowing that I believe in you, I know that you can beat this. I know because you are a human being and we are all adaptable. You learned to control your body before, and you can do it again. No, you're not as young as you once were, but after conception that's true for everybody. You've been overcoming adversity and climbing figurative mountains your entire life. There's no expiration date on the challenges of living. You don't get a free pass after a certain age. It would be best for your future outlook to avoid making excuses and get to work. After all, your dignity and self-respect are on the line here.

Actionable Recovery Strategies:
1. Ask yourself, how your choices have contributed to this stroke?
2. Seek out the answer to, "What can I do moving forward to avoid another stroke?"
3. Do your home therapies. No wiggle room, unless wiggling is part of your therapy.
4. Repetition is how you first gained control of your body as an infant and repetition is what will help you regain control. Try, repeat,

and try again.
5. Telling yourself that you can regain control by sitting around is denial. Unless navigating a river in Egypt is one of your long-term goals, avoid denial like the plague.

### *Chapter Three: Never Again!*

By now the healthcare professionals in your life have likely prescribed for you your own personal pharmacy. For now, you should follow their advice religiously. Take your pills as prescribed. Over time you may be able to find a more natural or dietary way of dealing with your stroke risk areas, but for the immediate future your best friend is the pharmaceutical industry. I am personally fond of essential oils. I find that they supplement my pharmaceuticals quite well. However, denial about your need for pharmaceuticals can be a recipe for another stroke. Statistically speaking, you have a better chance of having another stroke within five years of the last one.

It would also be my recommendation that you look for

effective ways to reduce your stress. Stress is a huge contributor to most strokes. I cannot emphasize this enough, try to avoid stress at all cost. To accomplish this, you need to examine every aspect of your life. If there is someone or something in your life that represents a significant amount of stress, they or it need to adjust or be banished from your life. I know that this sounds harsh and scary, you're probably becoming gradually dependent on everyone around you, and the thought losing someone is going to be difficult to accept. However, you had a stroke and now everything in your life has become difficult. You should avoid using people like a crutch, especially if they are contributing to an unhealthy environment, your life depends on your ability to change that environment to one that is stress free.

People are not the only source of stress in our lives. You are the cause of most of your own stress. You worry about things you cannot control (like what other people think of you). I have found worry to be a friend who leaves you feeling inadequate. I used to revel in my worrying. I believed that it was my worrying that made me great at my job and that worrying protected me and insulated me from harm. However, the truth was that my life was just a house of cards and eventually all the worry that kept everything in balance was a primary contributor to the whole structure collapsing under its own weight.

You will probably not be surprised to hear that the vast majority of Americans consume things that contribute to how much stress they feel. Caffeine, for example, can be a big culprit. Caffeine tricks your body into thinking that it has energy reserves that it doesn't have. As a result, you end up putting your body under stress, when it doesn't have the actual fuel to cope. It wears you down and exposes you to a variety of health issues. If you can't muster the needed energy more naturally then maybe you should let go of the activity that requires the energy.

Caffeine can also have a boomerang effect. While it may pick you up momentarily, it will drag you back down just as quickly and possibly amplify any depression or discouragement you are already feeling or are prone to feel. The primary goal here is to recover, not insulate your former lifestyle from change. The stroke has changed everything in your life and you need to change with it or

die trying to avoid change. The choice is really yours. Do you want control of your body back, or do you want to be pitied for the rest of your life? Thinking you have any other choice is just denial.
Recovery of your body and your dignity require all of your focus and determination. Don't lose sight of that.

Actionable Recovery Strategies:
1. Take the medications prescribed for you, until you discover effective natural and dietary alternatives.
2. Reduce stress, even if it means avoiding certain people.
3. Don't contribute to your own stress. Eat right and use caffeine judiciously.
4. Get used to change, stoke

is synonymous with change, and that's not a bad thing.
5. Do the work you've been assigned by your therapists or get used to being pitied. You are only pitiful when you give up or give in to old habits.

## *Chapter Four: Keep It in Perspective*

News flash, you didn't die, and if you believe that the universe has a purpose then it would be logical for you to believe that you have a purpose as in it. Consequently, since you're still with us there must be a reason you didn't die. If you're like me, you think that death would have been easier compared to this, but it didn't happen, so deal with it. Don't just sit around missing your old life and feeling sorry for yourself, self-pity is the worst kind of pity. It is the enemy within that slowly eats away at your resolve. You're still here for a reason and it's about time you figured out what that reason is. No wimping out and claiming that God or the universe is just trying to punish you. I'm sure that God and the universe have better things to do than to punish you. In the grand scheme of things you are puny and insignificant, but we don't live life on a grand scheme scale. In your small circle of the universe you are very significant and there is still something important for you to accomplish. It may just be that seeing you struggle to come back from this tragedy will inspire someone else to not give up. Maybe you don't believe that there is purpose in your survival, but looking for and finding one will be critical to your successful recovery.

Life is a precious gift, don't squander it on pointless skepticism. Get on your knees, tell God, the universe or whatever you chose to believe in, that you're sorry and then go do better. I know that God is forgiving and I assume that the universe is too. You're still here for a very specific reason. Passing it off as dumb luck doesn't change the reason why you're still here. When that higher power selected you to remain among us, it wasn't random, any more than picking up this book to read it was random. Things happen for a reason and that includes your stroke. From my own experience, I've found that my brain had adjusted to seeing life from a pessimistic standpoint, because pessimism was all it ever heard me express. So, when I felt that moving forward was hopeless, my brain agreed and I gave up. For reasons I can only speculate on, one miserable day I told myself, "There is nothing wrong with me, I am perfectly healthy and I have every reason to keep moving." After that, pushing past the pessimism became simple.

Meaning, for the rest of your life, is something you need to find. It requires effort on your part. It may take you the rest of your life to find meaning in your stroke and why it didn't kill you. However, finding that meaning is fundamental to your complete recovery. If you truly believe that you are an unwitting pawn in the great cosmic scheme of things then personal dignity should be meaningless to you and I am hard pressed to understand why you are even bothering to read anything.

I wrote this book to give you hope and encourage you to look to a higher power and for meaning and purpose in what has happened to you, and why you must follow the path to recovery. On that same note, I believe that in the absence of a belief in the existence of a higher power, hope is meaningless. In other words, I believe that belief in the existence of God can give life purpose and meaning and that hope is the pure expression of God's existence in our lives. It is hope in a brighter future and in an eternal Heaven that gives us courage to press forward and build that brighter tomorrow. I understand that there are some whose beliefs, or lack thereof, differ greatly from mine. To them I say, "Fine, write a book!"

Actionable Recovery Strategies:
1. There's a reason you're still alive. Look for that reason.
2. Everything happens for a reason. You will be surprised at what you find.
3. Even if it takes the rest of your life, figure out what that reason is. It may not be readily apparent, but it will present itself.

4. Hope is critical to your recovery. Look for reasons to hope. This is a critical step on the road you travel now.
5. Belief in a higher power brings hope. If you have no faith in a higher being, develop one. Nothing is more discouraging to me, and perhaps you as well, than the notion that, this life is all there is.

# Part II: Be Grateful [Coping with Anger]

## *Chapter five: Seriously? (Did this really just happen to me?)*

I know, it's easy for someone else to tell you to be grateful because they have no idea what it's like to recover from a stroke. However, I do know what it's like, and I'm still telling you to be grateful. Gratitude may be the furthest thing from your mind right now, but this is part of the whole change every stroke survivor needs to grow accustomed to seeking for and experiencing for themselves. Everything has changed and you need to change with it. That means your habits in how you respond to a crisis have to change as well. You have a lot to be grateful for. Let's start with the stroke. Since you're still alive, it could have been worse. It probably could have been worse and still left you alive. Worse would have meant a longer, harder recovery or no chance of recovery at all. Be grateful your stroke wasn't worse.

You probably have family around you willing to help and even if you don't you've been introduced to a new family, your therapy family who are willing to help. Either way you aren't alone in this struggle. The stroke recovery community is very large, and with 600,000 new members every year, it just keeps getting bigger. The perception that no one near you has any idea what it's like to recover from a stroke, is a minor inconvenience. They're probably at this moment searching the internet for information to help them be more empathetic, and there's tons of useful information out there. You may even want them to read this book, to get a better sense of things from a survivor's perspective.

You have experienced a disabling event and there are a whole host of government and other programs out there to help you. Your disability makes you special, so special that you are now lumped together with millions of others struggling with a physical or mental disability in a category called special needs individuals. There is an army of people out there looking for an opportunity to help you. Imagine what you could have accomplished before your stroke with so many resources at your disposal. Don't waste this opportunity. Reach out to all of these programs and take advantage of the abundant opportunities available to you. Thanks to a law in the U.S. called the Americans with Disabilities Act (A.D.A.), and similar laws around the globe, you will more easily be able access places like your doctor's office, the grocery store, businesses and community buildings. Since the A.D.A. was passed, the world has been re-engineered to accommodate you.

So, cheer up and look around at the opportunities your stroke has introduced you to. If you had suffered a heart attack, all of this abundance would not have been available to you. Of course, if you had suffered a heart attack, you wouldn't be disabled and likely wouldn't care. Be that as it may, you've been dealt the cards you have and you can play your hand as best as possible or you can give up and fold. However, until God or the universe decides you're done you still have to sit there until the game is over. If you do decide to fold, be prepared for the rest of the players to pity you as you pathetically sit there while the game goes on.

Actionable Recovery Strategies:
1. Everything about your life has changed, and you need to change your perspective along with it. Write down your perspective as it is right now and find a more positive way to view the same circumstances. Then follow that as your mission statement.
2. Despite how bad things seem, they could have been worse. Don't look for the worse, just accept that it exists.
3. You are one of approximately 800,000 people who had a stroke in the same year you did. You're not alone. Research your

local community of disabled individuals. They can inspire you and they need your inspiration.
4. Because of the prevalence of stroke and other disabling events, there are laws, government agencies, and other organizations ready to help you. You're not alone. Look into the resources available to you.
5. Cheer up, things are never as bad as they seem.

### *Chapter Six: Depression*

Depression is not the next stage of grief, but it seemed appropriate to address it at this point. Depression is a powerful side effect of stroke. It's important to understand what depression is. On a very simplistic level, I have found that post-stroke depression is your brain's reaction to the damage done by the stroke. It can cause you to feel tired, lethargic and unsettled. However, depression is a self-sustaining emotional state. What I mean is that depression feeds on itself. The more you give into it, the more it grows. Too often when we experience depression we go in search of a catalyst in our environment. We want to blame the depression on someone or something. Finding a cause for our depression only reinforces the depression itself, making it harder to shake loose from it. The healthiest approach to dealing with your depression is to just accept it for what it is, a physiological response to your stroke. Don't try to pin it on anyone or anything else. It just is what it is and it will usually pass. It may be re-occurring, and as discouraging as that is, it should still pass. Sometimes medication can help with this aspect of your recovery. However my experience has shown me that proper changes in diet will also help. The more you give your body to work with, the more it can accomplish for you. Right now, you're probably painfully aware that you need your body to do as much for you as possible. Shedding those extra pounds and feeding your body nutritiously gives your body the fuel it needs to perform at peak efficiency. The more efficient your body performs the less frustrated your brain will be. Reducing your brain's frustration level will result in a decrease in your moments of depression.

    Depression can be debilitating, it can rob us of our motivation to act responsibly in our own best interest. It can sometimes drive us to make very unhealthy choices. I can assure you that as powerful as your depression may be, you can still be in charge. Your depression can only take over, if you allow it to. As long as you maintain control, you can still make choices that will improve your situation and combat the depression. Don't listen to what the depression is telling you to do. It wants you to make choices that will feed and reinforce the depression, which is desperate to control you. By controlling you, it can get you to make poor choices and thereby maintain its existence. From my personal perspective, until you make positive choices that will reverse the depression, it will fight you every step of the way.

In a very real sense, as a stroke survivor, your brain is at war with itself. In this war your very life might be at stake. Your choices will determine the outcome of this war. It's highly likely that you made dietary and lifestyle choices which fueled or contributed to the depression in the first place. I can assure you, from personal experience, that accepting responsibility and choosing better will result in more favorable outcomes in the long term. For example, it will likely do you no good to take prescriptions to help you combat the depression and then turn around and eat or drink things that fuel the depression.

Don't tie your hands behind your back in this conflict. The depression needs your help to take over.

In my darkest hour, we had an interruption to our health insurance and I was without depression medication for a week. During this dark time, I wrote the following, "The world is an endless river of shit, and life is the process of wading across it." Interestingly, at the time I was still solidly on the side of "suicide is not an acceptable option." It wasn't until later, under less distressing circumstances that I calmly walked up to the boundary between suicide as/as not an option. I looked over that line. It seemed so tranquil there, but while the result looked appealing, I couldn't come to terms with the actual act. I knew that I would leave behind friends and family who would blame themselves for not being enough of a reason for me to stay and for not doing enough to help me cope. I assure you that you have similar people in your life. Imagine that you're driving a car and you are about to run a red light. What if you knew that you would be hit by another car and the good friend sitting next to you would end up crippled for the rest of his or her life. Would you still run that red light? Of course not. Well, suicide is that red light and others will be crippled by your choice. Don't do it.

    I agree with you on the point, "What business do your loved ones have blaming themselves when someone close to them decides to end it all?" Their guilt is entirely misplaced. In fact, I firmly believe that some people kill themselves as a means of punishing those around them. Both the attempt to lay guilt and the feelings of guilt are misplaced. Suicide is a personal choice, with very personal repercussions. If a loved one successfully commits suicide you are no more responsible for that outcome than you were responsible for the stroke that may have preceded it. Both suicide and stroke are responses to circumstances, and only the subject individual can control how they choose to respond. My own research into the subject has revealed that suicide is entirely motivated by the individual's intolerance for the situation they find themselves in. Granted, some people's lives can really suck, but suicide is rarely forced upon someone. Final statements, left by those who have attempted suicide often demonstrate that suicides are committed by people who have simply given up. They have chosen to hand over control to their depression. I have found, in my own case that depression is just a fantasy, bred from my reality, but it's still not real. It is a negative perspective on circumstances that could be, and usually are, interpreted differently by others who are observing your condition from the outside. Perception is very rarely reality, and your depression is only as powerful as you allow it to be.

Actionable Recovery Strategies:
1. Depression is just one more effect of the stroke. Don't try to blame it on someone or something around you. Just accept depression for what it is. A lie.
2. A war is raging in your head, between depression and your will to go on.

Depression can never win unless you allow it. Don't give in to depression.
3. Suicide is only possible if you choose to cross the line. There is nothing good on the other side. Don't be curious about what's on the other side. The grass isn't greener, if there even is grass.
4. Suicide is a permanent solution for a temporary problem. Just be a little more patient and circumstances will change.
5. You can always count on change. What you can never do is keep everything exactly the same. Don't resist

change, embrace it.

### *Chapter Seven: Therapy*

Even if you are bed or wheelchair bound, both of which I've been, you can still exert yourself and get the blood pumping through your body to carry the needed oxygen and nutrients to your brain. You can just lay there or sit there if you want, but I recommend that you give your brain what it needs to acquire and maintain a more positive outlook. It is a biological fact that the older we get the harder it is for us to learn. At some point, our brain decides that it is done learning and starts to rebel when we try to force it to. This is likely where you find yourself at now. Your brain no longer wants to learn, but you are still in control. You can choose to push yourself a little further. By repetitively performing the same tasks over and over again, you are forcing your brain to learn. If you are consistent and persistent, your brain will learn, whether it wants to or not.

Therapy is not a punishment. It is a tool for re-training your brain. You can allow your brain to act like a stubborn child and refuse to cooperate, or you can force your will onto your brain and demand that it obey you. You are in control until you give that control away. If you can remember, you had control before the stroke. Let your pre-stroke-self tell you how to regain and maintain control. How would you have responded to someone like your current self, before the stroke? I'm sure that you would have expected more from them. Likely you didn't always make the healthiest choices, but it's doubtful you were self-destructive. You are in charge and therapy is the only way you will be able to regain full control of your body. Commit yourself to it and stick with it until you have your body back.

Routine visits with your therapists to gauge your progress and adjust your home therapies will go a long way toward enhancing the effectiveness of your home therapy program. Don't put off meeting with your therapist because you've failed to do your therapies as prescribed. Accountability is key to your success in recovering your lost control. Failure to do the work, compounded with not holding yourself accountable will only make your situation worse. Be a grown-up and face the music. If you haven't done your therapies admit it. Saying you did your therapies when you didn't will only confuse the therapist who will be expecting different results. Your home therapy program is not just busy work. These are tried and true techniques for reprogramming your brain. Experience has shown your therapists that certain movements performed consecutively on a daily basis will yield specific results. Your active participation is key to your ultimate success.

One pitfall you may run into is that many people develop romantic feelings for their therapist. For a while this could even be advantageous, because you may be more motivated by a desire to please your therapist. However, it's all a fantasy and eventually reality will wake you up. It should come as no surprise to you that your therapist spends all day working with people as or more impaired than you. Why would they want to take one home with them? Ultimately, you have to decide that recovery is what you want. It needs to be what you're all about. Recovery requires dedication to home therapies. Without dedication you're looking at a permanent disability.

Actionable Recovery Strategies:
1. The older we get, the harder it is to learn, but hard is not the same as impossible. Don't get discouraged by the opportunity to learn. Learning keeps the brain active and pushes back Alzheimer's and dementia.
2. Your primary goal needs to be re-training your brain to re-learn what it has lost. You accomplish this through repetition.
3. Repetition of simple tasks is the best way to re-train your brain. Do your home therapies with full

confidence that they will lead you back to full recovery.
4. Do your home therapies. Do them, do them, do them.
5. Be honest with yourself and your therapist about how faithfully you are doing your home therapies. Lying or exaggerating your efforts will not help you recover and will confuse your therapist.

## Chapter eight: What You Don't Know

It's a hard concept to come to grips with, but you don't know what you no longer know. You've lost some sectors of your body's internal hard drive and there isn't an inventory for what's gone missing. You may still look and/or sound like you, so people will naturally assume that you are intact. Even those who know what you've been through are prone to forget occasionally and react badly when your deficiencies surface. It would be easier for everyone else to cope with if you had lost your memory entirely. Then they would have no expectations of you. Not knowing what you still remember puts others in an awkward position. They know that you don't want to be treated like you don't know anything, but they are continually reminded that you have forgotten a lot. It might actually be easier for you too, if you had forgotten everything. Then you wouldn't be so sensitive about being treated like a child; you wouldn't remember being treated like an adult. But imagine for a moment what that would be like. You don't remember who you or anyone else is. You may not even remember language. Imagine having to start all over from scratch with every aspect of your life.

    Not a pretty prospect, so be grateful that things aren't worse. At least you can communicate on some level. No, you're not 100%, but you aren't at zero either. Part of your body doesn't work quiet right, but it does still work and you can re-train it. Things could be so much worse, but they aren't and you have that to be thankful for.

Gratitude is going to be your best friend for the next few years. Gratitude lifts your mood and makes life worth living. If you are having trouble feeling grateful, try making a list of the things you think you should be grateful for. Read the list out loud to yourself every morning and any time you're feeling down. Say, "I am grateful for ..." and try to really mean it. Your brain listens to what you have to say, the more positive information you feed your brain, the more positively it will react to your situation. You may even want to start your day off with some positive affirmations like, "I am improving," "I am healthy," "I am strong," "I am capable," "I will conquer."

    Your brain is like a sponge, you get out what you put in. If you feed your brain negativity then negativity is what your brain will absorb and give you back in return. Avoid saying things like, "I can't," or "It's not possible," If something is difficult then say that instead. Nothing worth being good at ever came easy. No reasonable person expects for this process to not be challenging. You have a mountain to climb and gratitude is your oxygen. Without gratitude you'll never make it. Gratitude is the fuel that keeps you engaged. It influences everything you do and motivates you when you otherwise would just give up.

    I know it sounds counterintuitive to be grateful when so much has gone wrong, but it is your most critical therapy. Without it you're just a door stop, sitting around taking up space. I don't know you personally, but I do know that the list of things you have to be grateful for is longer than your arm. From this spectacularly beautiful world you live on to the individual elements that it's composed of. No matter where you live, you are surrounded with beauty and wonder, whether that beauty is natural or man-made it's all around you. If you are looking around the space where you spend the majority of your day, and you don't see beauty, you need to fix that. Hang up some pictures or paintings of the world's beauty. Even better, hang up pictures of places you plan to visit. Remind yourself that you are going to go there someday soon. Make specific plans and save your pennies. Tell others about your plans. Commit yourself to visiting these beautiful places. Set a date and work toward getting yourself ready physically, mentally and emotionally. Dare to dream. Dreams are what bring hope and hope can carry us through the most difficult of circumstances.

This is by no means a new concept. The Greek philosopher Epictetus said, "He is a wise man who does not grieve for the things which he has not, but rejoices for those which he has." You have lost a lot, but you can still be wise and focus on what you still have, which is also a lot.

Actionable Recovery Strategies:
1. The stroke completely erased the information in the affected sectors of your brain. The only way to get that information back, is to re-train your brain. Retraining means repetition.
2. Everyone around you is having to adjust to the fact that you've lost details due to the stroke. Try to be patient with

them as well. They have had to adjust their image of you, you should probably do the same.
3. Gratitude is your new go to friend. The more often you go there, the better your life will appear. Make a list of what you're grateful for, review it daily, and add to it regularly.
4. Surround yourself with beauty to remind you of what you're grateful for.
5. Plan a trip or other event to give yourself something to look forward to and work toward. Don't just sit around and mourn your losses.

### *Chapter nine: I'm done (This is the end of my rope)*

Everyone has their limits, we all reach a point at some time or another where we won't accept anything more. It's healthy and natural to set limits. What is not healthy or natural is to set unreasonable limits. When we set unreasonable limits we are begging for disappointment. Because of the stroke you have lost some of your freedom and autonomy. It's a difficult pill to swallow, but it is your reality for the time being. Freedom and autonomy are worth working hard for. Recovering from a stroke doesn't take tremendous physical exertion, but it does take monumental dedication and persistence. Giving up is not an option if you want to recover fully.

Anyone who has given up completely, and chosen to check

out of this life, had to cross the boundary between suicide being and not being an option. It should not be surprising to learn that you were born on the not-an-option side of that border. Human beings have natural survival instincts. As a species, we go to great lengths to ensure that we continue to exist, both individually and as a group. But some of us reach a point where we just can't take anymore and our instincts for survival become overwhelmed by our intolerance for our circumstances. At some point some people mentally and emotionally draw a line and say, "No more!"

Let's be perfectly clear on one point, suicide is an emotional response not a logical decision. No matter what your circumstances are right now, they are temporary. Everything changes. In fact, change is one thing you can truly count on. So tolerating your current circumstances is a temporary state. Your circumstances will change in a relatively short period of time. In fact, if you find your situation to be intolerable, I encourage you to catalog the specific intolerable issues and then check them off as they disappear.

     Suicide is a permanent solution to a temporary problem. It's excessive and unnecessary. You don't need to end your life in order to cope better with your situation. You just need to humble yourself and be more accepting of the hand you've been dealt. Instead of saying that you can't take it anymore, focus on what is right and positive in your life. Look for beauty, friendship and family. Cling desperately to the things you can be grateful for. Instead of wasting time planning your own death, make plans to take a trip. Do something different. Stop focusing on what's fair. On the greatness scale, fair is pretty far down the list. Fair is not something to shoot for. Instead, change up your routine, if for no other reason than to just be different. If you don't like your life the way it is, change something. Since change is something thing you can truly count on then embrace change. Be purposefully changing on a continual basis. If the old you was steady and reliable, make the new you spontaneous and unpredictable. Yes, the people in your life will complain, because their own routines depend on you being dependable and predictable, but they will just have to get over it. Your survival instincts are telling you to embrace change and that's what you're going to do. You have nothing to offer anyone else if all you want is to be dead.

I understand the appeal of death, I have wanted to be dead for most of my life. But wanting death and making it happen are dramatically different things. Again, you're still here for a reason. Don't cash in your chips when the game is just getting interesting. If your life was a movie, the stroke is just a plot twist. It's an inciting moment, a catalyst for change. Suddenly, the main character is forced to choose between fighting and giving up. Come on, you know you want the protagonist of your own movie to fight. Fighting is much more interesting and exciting than giving up. Do you really want your movie to end with the hero giving up? Fight! Fight with everything you have inside you. Change is going to happen anyway, take charge and own the change. This story's ending hasn't been written yet. The stroke wasn't the climax, you decide what the climax be. The climax could be something athletic, something organizational, something creative, or something artistic. The climax could also be something musical or literary. From this point forward it's your job to write the climax for the movie of your own life. Shoot for something spectacular and inspirational, I personally look for that in a good story. Going from where you are now to inspirational may seem like a huge leap, but trust me, every day you keep plugging away at your recovery you are inspiring someone.

    In August of 2014, the world was shocked to learn that Robin Williams, one of the most successful comedians of all time, had hung himself. It was hard to process that information. By most people's standards, Robin had everything to live for. He had piles of money, fame, and children who loved him. He was adored the world over, and we all welcomed him into our homes in films like Disney's Aladdin and Dead Poet's Society. Now he joins a growing list of amazing people who checked out too soon. Some people are so confused by his decision that they are convinced he was murdered. I suspect that there will always be theories as people try to make sense of a seemingly senseless act. Oh, I'm sure that Robin had reasons that made perfect sense to him at the time, but when you leave the rest of the world scratching their heads, your reasons are not very convincing. In fact most people will disagree with your reasoning, if you make that choice. The reasons only make sense when seen through the lens of depression. That's why no one should ever be permitted to make that choice. Perspective is warped by depression and what you perceive as reality is really a delusion. Reality is actually quite different from what you perceive when you're depressed. If you find your situation intolerable, just keep telling yourself that it isn't real. It won't be a lie. Depression is the lie.

Actionable Recovery Strategies:
1. Set healthy limits. Chose achievable goals and be dedicated to accomplishing them.
2. Do something different or be someone different. Change is reliable, it will always happen. Keep yourself open to changing along with your circumstances. There is no

advantage to trying to go back to who you were. Move on to a new and better you.
3. The finality of death is appealing, but suicide emotionally and psychologically cripples the loved ones you leave behind. If you feel that suicide is your only option, decide which of your loved ones you want to cripple in the process and then don't.
4. Depression is a perception, not a reality. The best way to change your reality is to change your perception. Make a list of what contributes to your feelings of depression, then tell yourself, I will no longer believe each lie."

5. Telling yourself that depression isn't real is not a lie. Depression is the lie. Depression's vulnerability is that it isn't true. Call it out and see it for what it is.

### *Chapter ten: Win the Race*

As I sit here writing on this edition , I am coming up on the five year anniversary of my stroke. Mine was a right brain stroke, so the left side of my body was affected. Immediately following the event I had no movement in my left side. For all intents and purposes half of my body was dead. I had also been a very type "A" personality before the stroke, stressing and worrying about everything. While I have gradually regained most of the control over my left side, my personality appears to be forever changed. In fact, my wife sometimes accuses me of not caring about anything and my former employer commented several times that I wasn't the same person, a perspective which later resulted in my termination.

I have no wish to compare my recovery experience to yours, and you must feel free to do the same. I only want to share with you my experiences, in the hopes that something might help you along your way. I have gone from being completely immobile and bed ridden, to getting around in an electric wheelchair, to completing a 5K race two years post-stroke. In fact it was during that race that the idea for this book came to me. I am a writer and many people had been encouraging me to write a book about stroke recovery, but I saw how many books on the subject already existed and I thought that there was really nothing I could offer that wouldn't just be a rehash of the same tired material. I continued to push back against the encouragement until the thought occurred to me, during my participation in that particular event, that personal dignity is a critical aspect of how we view ourselves through the eyes of others. However stroke affects dignity the way it affects everything else, it takes a sledge hammer to it. At least I felt that dignity had been ripped away from me, and I was helpless to get it back. Then, as others told me how inspired they were by me, I realized that dignity was not the problem, but rather how I defined dignity. Suddenly a book seemed possible where before it had seemed impossible. Don't discount the possibility that you might have an epiphany down the road and your whole perspective on a subject might change. Again, change is one thing you can always count on.

I'm sure that in the immediate aftermath of my stroke, I couldn't see myself competing in a 5K foot race. In all fairness, competing is probably too strong of a word. I walked most of the way, jogged a little, and came in last. No one else's placement in the rankings was ever in any jeopardy. It took me one hour and fifteen minutes to complete the three mile course. That puts my average speed at just above two miles per hour. My gut told me that I was embarrassing myself, that I was going so slow and taking so long to complete a course that, before the stroke, I could have completed it in far less time, but as a result of my perseverance and determination several people shared with me, after the race, how inspired they were by my effort. If you want to maintain or re-claim your dignity, be inspirational.

    Since the stroke, if we go somewhere that requires a lot of walking, my wife would always insist that I be in a scooter or wheelchair. However, two days after the 5K we walked into Walmart and she didn't even hint at the scooters. Score! I had been desperate to find something to improve the way my wife perceived me, in the aftermath of the stroke, which was generally feeble and prone to fall. However, anything that elevated her perception of me, I was happy to take. I had been inadvertently making a classic mistake. Many of us tend to believe that we are who others perceive us to be, but it's never that simple. You are complex in a myriad of ways. No two people see you exactly the same and you are so much more than what you let anyone see. Since your stroke, who you are now is an even bigger mystery to others. Yours is not the only world that was rocked by this stroke. As you show others your persistence and determination, you get bonus dignity points. There are no written rules for how to cope with stoke, for you or for them. Everyone is doing what they can to feel their way across what must look like a minefield to the outside observer and feels like one to you.

    Your expectations of others, and how well those expectations are met, will have a huge impact on how well you navigate this mine field. Give people the benefit of the doubt. You'll be happier and so will they. There is no conspiracy to keep you disabled or to make your life miserable. If you're miserable, it's because that's what you want to be. Don't blame others for the fact that you choose misery. Happiness is also a choice, now go make that choice instead.

Actionable Recovery Strategies:
    1. If you want to maintain,

or re-claim your dignity, inspire others. It's not hard, you already do it without thinking about it.
2. You are more than what you allow others to see. Their perception of you is not your reality. Inspire them and they will see you differently.
3. There are no rules for how to cope with a stroke, for you or for those around you. Everyone is just trying to figure it out, the best way they know how. Be as patient and understanding as you want to be treated.
4. Managing your expectations will aid in your recovery and your relationship with others. Expect from yourself only what is reasonable and

accomplishable.
5. If you're miserable it's because you choose to be. Choose differently.

**Part III: Work Your Butt Off
[There is no Negotiating Here]**

### *Chapter eleven: Start Every Day with a Plan*

Structure is important to your overall success. If you think that you can take a free form, or shoot from the hip, approach to stroke recovery you are deluding yourself. The only way to re-gain control of your body is to be consistent. Repeat this over and over to yourself, "I will try and try again." You can't afford to lose sight of the big picture. Your main goal is to recover completely, and if you put in the necessary effort, you will succeed. While you will likely never be back to the old you, you will be a better, healthier you. A new you with better habits, a better outlook and perspective on life, and a greater capacity to overcome problems in the future.

When you get out of bed in the morning, make a list of things to accomplish in your day. Don't be unrealistic. You have limitations and pretending you don't or ignoring them will not make them go away. Understand you capabilities and your inabilities and factor that into any daily goals you make. Your list should be achievable under favorable circumstances. That means that on a "good day" you can get everything done.

So, what if today isn't a good day? Bad days will happen. Just accomplish what you can and save whatever's left for the next day. Don't beat yourself up because you couldn't accomplish everything, but be honest with yourself. Did you try your best? If you didn't then just try harder the next day.

Your goals should be three things, achievable, worthwhile and satisfying. You don't want to set a goal for yourself to accomplish something that you know you're going to put off as long as possible. However, if it needs to be done regardless, then bite the bullet and get it done first. Your list of daily goals should be self-motivating. If your goals are things you know you can do, they're worth your time and effort, and you will derive some personal satisfaction from accomplishing them then you will be far more likely to complete your list. Any goals that are in anyway unenjoyable should be accomplished early in the day when you're still fresh, rested and energetic, which brings us to the next subject, "home therapies".

Actionable Recovery Strategies:
    1. Structure is important. You can't make up recovery as you go. Perform the tasks assigned to you by your

therapist.
2. Full recovery is not only possible, it's probable based on your attitude and perspective. You're daily home therapy commitment determines your level of recovery.
3. Make lists and keep a record of what you accomplish. Looking back and seeing your progress can give you courage to press on.
4. Do what you can, and save anything else for the next day. Make your goals reasonable and achievable.
5. Tackle the harder items on your list first.

### *Chapter Twelve: Gettin'er Done! (You've got this.)*

As we discussed previously, therapy is not a punishment. Therapy is the tool you will use to regain control of your body. Sitting around just reading, watching T.V. and surfing the internet will not restore your body to its former glory. However, you can still do those things as long as you are incorporating your home therapies at the same time. Your therapist has likely given you some gross and some fine motor skill exercises to perform for a specific amount of time each day. They generally don't require sight or a lot of concentration. Which means that at the same time you can otherwise engage your mind. In fact, I strongly encourage you to keep your brain occupied as much as possible. I would also encourage you to take steps to make your therapy time a treat. Put off streaming that show you love until you are ready to do your therapies or plan your therapies around when the show normally airs. That way the show is like a little reward for sticking to your therapy schedule. Don't, and this is important, don't get so engrossed in what you're watching or reading that you forget to do the therapies. Be sure to reward yourself for doing the work, but don't fall into the trap of rewarding yourself without doing the work. That path leads to permanent disability.

Repetition has long been known as an effective learning tool. In fact, there are a few very famous quotes surrounding the concept:

Norman Vincent Peale - "Repetition of the same thought or

physical action develops into a habit which, repeated frequently enough, becomes an automatic reflex."

Reggie Jackson - "A baseball swing is a very finely tuned instrument. It is repetition, and more repetition, then a little more after that."

Dale Carnegie - "Learning is an active process. We learn by doing. Knowledge that is used sticks in your mind."

Aristotle - "What we have to learn to do, we learn by doing."

You are one of about 800,000 people who had a stroke in the year your stroke occurred. Whether your stroke was mild or severe, your therapists have a plan to get you back to whatever normal was before the stroke, if at all possible. That plan is mostly dependent on you. Your therapists can show you what normal movement looks and feels like, and they can recommend certain movements you can practice at home, but if you don't put in the work, recovery will not be complete. If you had a child who was anticipated to perform a piano piece before dignitaries in a month, you would sit that child down and lay out a practice schedule that would ensure that they performed well. Like the old joke says, "How do you get to Carnegie Hall?", "Practice, practice, and more practice." In this case, you are the child and you have a deadline. Five years after your stroke, you will not be expected to make much more of an improvement. So, you have five years to reclaim your body and the clock is ticking. It's remarkable how fast five years can go by and you're going to need every second of that time. Don't kid yourself that you've got plenty of time. The time is now, and the work has to be done by you. No one else can recover from this stroke for you. Your therapists are there to guide you and advise you, but you have to be the one to make it happen. Practice, practice, and keep on practicing.

Actionable Recovery Strategies:
1. Your home therapies are your ticket to restoring full use of your body and mind. Do your home therapies.
2. If you use methods to distract your mind during your home therapy, be sure to maintain focus on the primary goal.
3. Repetition is the key, it is

how you've always trained your brain and it is the only way you will be able to re-train it.
4. Consider what you would expect from you before the stroke. It would be inconsistent for you to expect less of an effort from yourself now.
5. This is not the time to sit on your hands. Now is the time to act.

### *Chapter Thirteen: It's No Picnic (Recovery is work)*

You're going to get tired, you're going to get frustrated, and you might even get angry. Oh well! Life goes on, and the extent to which you will be able to keep up is entirely in your hands. Is it hard? Yes. Is it fair? Probably not. Will you grow tired and bored of your therapies? Yes. Will you hate or at least resent your therapists? Sometimes. Are you alone? Absolutely not! Everyone in your life and society as a whole has a vested interest in helping you get better. If you are left with any deficiencies after five years, we all have to deal with it. If you don't fully recover then everywhere you go people will be forced to make accommodations for you. You are not a burden. Most people will help you willingly and gladly, but occasionally you will meet that very unpleasant person who is too busy, too much in a hurry, or too irritable to be bothered by you. Don't take it personally, they treat everyone, they don't need something from, that way.

As the saying goes, "If life gives you lemon's, make lemonade." Well there are no shortage of lemons in your life now. Won't a tall, cold glass of fresh lemonade be refreshing? Well, lemonade doesn't make itself. "You've got to squeeze a lot of lemons, if you want to make lemonade." Your work is cut out for you. Your therapists have mapped out the path back to full functionality, if that's even possible. You can either follow the map or wander around on your own. If you chose to wander, don't be surprised when five years rolls around and you are still severely limited.

If you've already hit the five year mark, don't give up. Your progress will be slower after five years, but the situation isn't hopeless. The effect of repetition is incontrovertible. You can still improve, but you'll have to take my advice as gospel and be hyper dedicated and uber-vigilant. Take whatever your therapists tell you to do or told you to do in the past and double it or triple it. You're going to feel like a slave to therapy, but if you truly want to recover more of your lost mobility, you have no other option. If you haven't crossed the five year threshold, my advice to you is the same. Work today like it's your last chance. Don't focus on progress or the lack thereof, I promise you that, if you put in the work then the progress will come.

In the immortal words of

Lynn Anderson "...I never promised you a rose garden." This is serious work and it requires a serious and dedicated mind. Your brain is what got damaged and it should not seem ironic to you that your mind is where we're putting all of the responsibility for your recovery. When I was a kid, I had a t-shirt that read, "Do a good job and what do you get? More work!" Of course, as a child, I saw "work" as a four letter word. Now, with all of these recommendations (work) you probably feel that, on top of everything else, I'm just dumping a huge pile of crap on you.

Crap has many defining characteristics, but perhaps its most endearing quality is that it helps things to grow. Right now, you need to grow. Consider yourself encouraged. The seeds have already been planted and now they need to be nourished and nurtured, so that they take root and emerge from the soil and the fertilizer to grow tall and strong and bear fruit. Sorry, I keep mixing my metaphors, so yes, on top of everything else, you're a gardener now. The list of things you need to do is long and most of those things are mundane, repetitive and unspectacular. The results of completing that list, however, are quite spectacular. From bed ridden to running races in less than two years is no small thing. Obviously, I can't promise you that you will have the same results, but it's worth the try. Your results will be as unique as you and your stroke are. The limits of your recovery are what you make of them. The British Prime Minister, Winston Churchill, said during the Second World War, "Never give up! Never surrender." That is my best advice to you. There is no dignity in accepting defeat. It is the struggle that defines us and reveals our dignity. Climb that hill and don't stop climbing until you're safely on the other side.

Actionable Recovery Strategies:
1. You will get tired and bored of your therapies. Push past that and stay focused.
2. It is in everyone's best interest that you fully recover. You know you need help, so let others help.
3. The more time goes by, the more you need to ramp up your efforts. If twenty repetitions a day is good, fifty is even better. Push yourself.
4. Nurture the seeds of recovery that you have already planted. Nurture

them and they will grow.
5. You have a hill to climb, better get started.

### Chapter Fourteen: "When Will It Ever End?" I'm sorry that sounded an awful lot like a complaint.

At one point, about two years into my recovery, in a fit of frustration, I just stopped doing my home therapies. This hiatus lasted six months and at the end of it, I had lost most of the progress I had made over the previous year. Please note, I didn't lose everything, just the most advanced elements of my recovery. Your recovery will happen in stages. Stage one – is gross motor skills. Stage two – is fine motor skills. Stage three – is targeted fine tuning of what you already have back. Stage four – as we have already discussed is maintenance. It has been my experience and observation that recovery takes a lifetime. You may have become very critical of your body and even when you regain full functioning, you will continue to tweak it in a quest for greater perfection. What you are attempting is the very definition of body building. Even if you can only lift ten pounds, or take two steps, you're a body builder. You are building and re-building a fully functional body from what may have once been lifeless lumps of flesh, immediately after the stroke.

    You aren't a sprinter, you're running cross country now, and there are miles and miles left to run. You can't see the finish line from here, because there really isn't one. You win this race by continuing to run. Of course there are mile markers you can use to calculate your progress with. You've probably already passed several of them. Look back at what you've already accomplished, but don't stop to look. Keep moving and make the most of the time you've been given. I know it may be hard to accept, but this stroke is—a gift. An opportunity to do something truly inspirational before you leave this existence. What you make of this opportunity is entirely up to you.

Now, back to this movie about yourself that you're writing, directing, and starring in. Obviously it has an end, but it ends with all of us missing you, because you're gone. Don't be in a hurry to jump to the end. The best parts of a movie are usually in the middle and toward the end. The actual ending of most movies is anticlimactic, sappy or dull. Enjoy writing every moment now, while you still can. It will all be over soon enough. For now, there are still chapters left to write. Make them memorable.

Actionable Recovery Strategies:
1. Stop counting down the days. You're in this for the long haul. Even when you get to a recovery stage you are comfortable with, that stage will need to be maintained. Accept therapy as your new way of life.
2. You are a body builder. I don't recommend that you sign up for any competitions, but you should be proud of what you're trying to accomplish, it reveals your character and your abundant dignity. Great work!
3. Recovery is a long process. Put on your cross country running shoes and stretch really well before

you hit the road running.
4. You've already passed significant mile markers in this run. Praise and reward yourself for all of your hard work.
5. Remember, this is your story, don't cut yourself out of the best scenes. Be present in your own story.

# Part IV: Something For Everyone [Advice For Others in Your Life]

### *Chapter Fifteen: Stroke Widow*

*This is my first attempt to define stroke. It made my wife cry. (Quotes were taken from the film Invasion of the Body Snatchers, Sunset Studios, 1956)*

*"The words, the gesture, the tone of voice, everything else is the same, but not the feeling."*

When your spouse has a stroke and doesn't die, they congratulate you saying that it could have been worse. It has been my experience, however, that in most cases your spouse did die, but they let you keep the body. The person inhabiting your spouse's body may look like your spouse, they may sound like your spouse, they may even have most of your spouse's memories and act like your spouse occasionally, but surprise, it turns out that they are decidedly not your spouse. I know it sounds like a scene out of <u>Invasion of the Body Snatchers</u>, but it's quite real and all too common.

*"Is this an example of your bedside manner, doctor?"*

The physical or public aspect of your spouse is challenging enough. This previously competent, confident and independent adult has suddenly become like a toddler. He or she needs to learn to walk, talk, and to hold things in their stroke affected hand. They have trouble remembering from one minute to the next and require constant reminding and encouragement. They are likely stubborn, typically because they remember who and how they were before the stroke, and they resent the tendency on everyone's part to treat them like they're an imbecile. Perhaps worst of all, it is likely that your spouse is in denial of their own condition. They may acknowledge that the stroke occurred and the fact that they have physical limitations is undeniable, but they may balk at the idea that they are suffering any diminished mental capacity. Unfortunately, in this, as the caregiving spouse, you are likely sabotaged by the professionals who are treating your spouse. Their goal is to provide encouragement and emotional support as your loved one struggles to regain the full use of their limbs and speaking ability. They are probably full of all kinds of supportive, validating and uplifting phrases. However, chances are great that they didn't know your spouse before the stroke, so their validation may generate a false sense of normalcy in the mind of your spouse. These professionals deal with every degree of stroke damage, therefore the bar that they are measuring your spouse by may be very low. If this is the case then any level of cognition or physical responsiveness is viewed by them as cause for celebration. They may also ascribe to the notion that encouragement is the most effective motivator, which may or may not be true. An equal number of people in this world, primarily task or purpose driven individuals, are motivated by constructive criticism. A never ending string of compliments and other encouragements may actually have a dampening effect on your spouse. Of course, I'm no psychologist, so take that for what it's worth.

*"I'd hate to wake up in the morning and find out you weren't you."*

While everything related to your spouse's stroke is linked to the brain, very few people are cognizant of the changes that have taken place there. They see the physical disabilities associated with the brain damage caused by the stroke, or rather is the stroke, but they don't know the extent to which it has changed your spouse. Essentially, the stroke affected person in bed next to you, or in the next room, may very well be a stranger and not the person you married. While it is true that we each change over time and twenty years later anyone's spouse is not the person they married. However, in that case you would have had twenty years to acclimate to those changes. Now take an equal or greater amount of change and imagine it happening overnight. Ideally, as their spouse you would be able to say, "Okay, this is who I am married to now," and move on. That, is a little like asking someone to accept an arranged marriage. Whether someone was born in a culture where arranged marriages are the norm or not, the prospect is frightening. They're being asked to commit themselves to someone they may no longer know. As the spouse of someone recovering from a stroke, you may find yourself struggling with issues of, "will you like them?", and the uncertainty of, "will they like you?" In many respects, as the spouse, you may be starting a new relationship, but strangely enough with someone who you have many years of shared experience with; experiences you both remember in detail. It is likely that this near stranger isn't aware of the extent to which they have changed and may be confused by your reactions to their behavior. Trust is a huge issue. Trust is something that develops over time. Now, suddenly, the person you used to trust has been taken by the stroke and in their place is a person who behaves differently and may even think differently. The trust you had in your spouse before the stroke may be gone. Your stroke affected spouse will likely not immediately understand why you no longer trust them. From their perspective, they haven't changed and the only thing they see changing is how you perceive and react to them. Over time, however, the extent of the change caused by the stroke will become increasingly more obvious to them as well. Patience, it's a word you probably hear a lot and you're likely getting sick of it, but over time, and with proper and frequent therapy, the personality change issues, as with most effects of the stroke, will work themselves out.

*"The mind is a strange and wonderful thing. I'm not sure it will ever be able to figure itself out."*

In the meantime, as the spouse of a person recovering from a stroke, you may feel very much alone. For all intents and purposes, your companion may have died. That would make you a widow or widower and you may have been left to babysit and be the primary caregiver of a very large and somewhat familiar infant; the most stubborn and uncooperative baby you've ever cared for. He or she is likely extremely dependent but struggling daily to maintain a sense of independence that babies should have no memory of. Just as you would with other toddlers, you should set limits for the protection of your stroke affected spouse and that of others. The stroke affected spouse will likely blanch at the limitations you impose and, like smaller toddlers will fail to understand the need for these limitations and try to find ways around them, this isn't a bad thing. Problem-solving is a higher brain or executive brain function and you want to encourage that. However, you will have to be extra vigilant. Unlike smaller toddlers, your spouse has a lifetime of experience to draw from; assuming their long term memory is still intact. Even if their memory loss is severe, their instincts may not have been affected and they may still be able to feel their way through to a solution. So, be ever watchful.

*"I can't do it, I can't, can't, can't go on."*

Most importantly, as the primary caregiver of someone recovering from a stroke, take care of yourself. Caring for a stroke victim can be emotionally and physically draining. Don't let yourself get run down. As the main source of support for someone recovering from a stroke, schedule out some time for yourself. Leave your stroke affected spouse in someone else's care for a while and get away. You'll be no good as a caregiver if you are burned out. Take a page out of my personal experience. As a result of my stroke, I was no longer able to perform my job. My wife had to get a job, and still, we took a hefty pay cut. On top of working full time and worrying constantly about money, she was worrying about me, my welfare and my continued progress, as well as the three children still at home, she also had community and church auxiliary responsibilities. Her load was heavy. I tried to help, but would often just make things worse. She was managing, but it was starting to burn her out. Finally, she took some time for herself; time to think, to relax and enjoy catching up with old friends. Me time is not just a good idea, but for you who care for a stroke victim, I firmly believe it's imperative.

### **Caregiver Strategies:**
1. Just because your spouse's body is still alive doesn't mean they're the same person they were before the stroke. Focus on what still makes them the person you loved.
2. Committing to this new person may seem like agreeing to an arranged marriage. That's focusing on the negative. Be positive, You need it and so do they.
3. Your stroke affected spouse is likely not aware

of how they have changed. From their perspective the only change may be the way you react toward them. Give them time to see the truth, but don't continually throw it in their face.
4. These personality changes may be temporary and can work themselves out over time. However, prepare yourself for the possibility that some changes are permanent.
5. As the primary caregiver of someone recovering from a stroke, make sure you take time for yourself. Don't let yourself get burned out.

## Chapter Sixteen: The Well Intentioned Spouse

We all want things that we can't have. Sometimes it's a husband or wife exactly the way we want them. We are not satisfied for nature to take its course. We want what we want and we want it now. You would think that over the many years of recorded history that nature would have cured us of this malady, but instead some of us have developed it into an art form, mastering ever more effective means of manipulation and psychological torture to extract the behavior we want.

However, it has been my observation that individuaevolution occurs when someone decides to change. Not from one species to another (inter-species evolution), but one personality type to another or one behavioral pattern to another (Intra-species evolution). They may have changed to adapt to a sudden shift in their environment brought on by a sudden change of employment, economic status or medical condition. But like coal under intense pressure becomes a diamond, they gradually change. This evolutionary process need not have a positive result to be valid. Its only purpose is to help the individual adapt and survive under the new environmental conditions. However, my personal experience has taught me that the one thing it "must be" is voluntary.

    I have observed that anyone can change their behavior temporarily to avoid pain or achieve a purpose, but such temporary change does not constitute evolution. Evolution requires a willingness to completely give oneself over to the change. In that way, the change is fully integrated into the individual and there is no part of them that rebels against it. Evolution doesn't occur unless the change is complete.

    I have learned that, when we seek to force change on an individual, the most we can hope for is temporary change, because some part of the individual continues to resist the change. No matter how unpleasant we make life for them, they refuse to fully embrace the change and therefore the change is not complete and evolution does not occur. Once the environment changes back, or the new environmental factor is removed the individual reverts back into their former state. Hence the old saying, "When the cat's away, the mice will play." It would appear from this saying that the preferred state for mice is playful and that the cat inhibits this behavior. However, the cat has not caused the desired evolution in the mice, because the moment the cat leaves the mice revert to their former playful behavior.

Bringing this back around to the subject of stroke recovery. Your loved one has experienced a powerful change physiologically and psychologically. The stroke has affected them in ways that may not have even surfaced yet. Those changes only become evolutionary when your spouse accepts them as permanent and fully gives themselves over to it. For example, having been a high stress individual in my pre-stroke life, I am fully aware of what stress feels like and what it can do to you. I know how my body reacts to stress and you couldn't pay me to have anything to do with it now. I have fully and completely rejected stress in all its forms. Therefore my evolution to a stress free life is complete. I have not only rejected stress on an emotional and psychological level, I have rejected it physiologically and philosophically. Stress used to keep me sharp and on top of things. It insulated me from the embarrassment caused by stupid little mistakes. Alright, I'll just say it, I was nearly perfect. But seriously, worrying about every little detail is tedious and exhausting. At this moment I can't imagine what was so appealing about it. I do remember the way people treated and responded to me. It was much different. But if to get that level of respect back I have to take the stress back with it. No way, no how.

    As the spouse of someone who has had a stroke, your loved one may be experiencing a similar evolutionary process. It can be a good thing, but if it's not, it will only become permanent when they fully embrace it and give themselves over to it. Remember this is a voluntary process. You can't prevent it. You can only influence it. Tread softly, you don't know where they are in their evolution, if you are too obvious with your intentions, you may be what pushes them over the edge. Here's where the art of manipulation, some of us have mastered, can come in handy. To short circuit their evolution, you need to get them to see why it's a bad thing. There is something about what they are evolving away from that is so distasteful that it has prompted this shift. If you want to prevent this change from becoming permanent, you might want to consider trying to figure out what they are evolving away from and try to alter their perspective of it. In my experience, people don't evolve toward something so much as they evolve away from something else. Like my aversion to stress.

As the innocent bystander in this drama, you can play a pivotal role. The key is to not appear manipulative or to have an agenda other than to support your loved one's happiness. Ultimately that's all this is for them, the pursuit of happiness. Whatever is motivating this change may simply be a problem of perspective. As their spouse, you are in the best position to help them change their perspective. If someone had gotten me to appreciate stress and view it as my friend, following my stroke, I might still be me. Of course I might also be dead. Change isn't always a bad thing.

## **Actionable Recovery Strategies:**
1. Change can be temporary or evolutionary. Don't misjudge change as automatically a bad thing.
2. Evolution happens when someone gives themselves over to change fully and completely. Embrace change and help your spouse to embrace it as well.
3. The effects of evolution can be minimized by identifying the source. It's the thing they are moving away from. Help them to see their path.
4. Tread carefully, if you are too obviously manipulative you might push them over the edge.
5. Evolution is all about happiness. As long as your loved one believes that you only want their happiness, they will allow you to

influence them, but be sincere.

## Chapter Seventeen: Stroke from your young child's perspective

I have discovered that, to a young child with a parent who had a stroke, mom or dad just out of nowhere started to act funny. Age plays an important role in their greater grasp of the mechanics of a stroke and some will be more astute than others. Still, the child's relationship to you is much different from that of your spouse, so their perspective of the changes is different. What they know is that their parent is sick, which is upsetting to young children. On top of it disrupting the schedule they have come to rely on, they naturally start thinking about death and that the parent may not always be there for them. In an intriguing article on the Children's Hospital of Philadelphia website called <u>A Child's Concept of Death,</u> The author explains how children in different developmental age groups deal with illness and death. It is perhaps ironic that preschool aged children interpret illness as a punishment for something they did. So, if you're looking for a reason why you tend to think that God or the universe is punishing you, there you go, pre-programmed from birth. You developed that perspective before you were five years old. But you need not listen to or take advice from your three or four year old self. You've developed much better coping skills in more recent years.

    This stroke didn't just happen to you. It happened to everyone around you. It didn't just rock your world. Yes, you did take the brunt of it, and you shoulder the lion's share of the issues, but it's not all about you. Everyone's life, in the family and close to you has been impacted and inconvenienced. It's important that you acknowledge that and remember it when you're feeling put upon or neglected. Everyone in the family was impacted and is coping with it as best way they can.

Children are by nature very "me" centric. Not to say that they are naturally selfish, but they are overly preoccupied with themselves. The stroke has now taken the focus off of them and put it on you. If anyone has cause to feel neglected it's them. I'm not suggesting that perspective is valid, mind you. However, from their perspective some, if not most of the attention that used to be focused on them has shifted to you. It is perfectly natural that they should be experiencing some resentment toward you for that. You shouldn't feel guilty or ashamed of this, just be aware of it.

    Experience has shown me that because children are accustomed to being asked to help they are often willing and eager to do so; especially if it shifts more attention toward them. I recommend that you involve your children in your therapy and in retrieving things for you, so that you don't place yourself in a precarious position unnecessarily. Your former, independent self may balk at the concept of relying on your children to handle menial tasks for you, but do it anyway. It's good for them and better for you. It will help them to feel more important and involved and it gives them a greater awareness of your new needs. You are no less of a parent because you have needs. I must warn you, however, that there is a danger that they may begin to see you and treat you as a peer. This is especially true, if your spouse or other adults are treating you like a child. To help stem this tide, I suggest that you be open with the children about what's going on. Explain to them how recovering from a stroke and learning like a baby can be similar. Be the expert on your own stroke recovery. Children are capable of understanding more than most adults give them credit for. Use smaller words that are easily accessible to them and explain the same thing multiple times in different ways, Answer their questions honestly. The greater their understanding of your situation, the less scary it will be, and their ability to empathize with

you will be enhanced.
## **Actionable Recovery Strategies:**
1. Your stroke didn't happen only to you. Everyone around you has been affected and is doing their best to cope. Be patient.
2. Your children have a much greater capacity to understand and empathize than you may think. Don't talk down to them.
3. Be open with them about what has happened to you and what you have to do to get it all back.
4. Children are primarily focused on themselves and they expect everyone around them to be similarly focused on them. Make an effort to involve them.
5. Don't be afraid or reluctant to ask them for help. It shifts some attention back their

way, which they like, and they'll probably be willing to help. You do need the help.

### *Chapter Eighteen: A script for explaining stroke to small children*

[Script] As you know, Mommy or Daddy has had a stroke. A stroke happens when a part of the brain doesn't get enough blood and stops working. Since the brain is where you keep everything you know, if a part of it stops working then you will forget things. Sometimes you forget people's names or who they are. Sometimes you forget how to move or control a part of your body. Whatever has been forgotten has to be relearned again. Learning takes time; especially re-learning how to move your body. The only way to re-teach the body how to move is by making it do the same things over and over again. This is called repetition, and we use repetition to help our brain learn and re-learn how to move properly.

Because mommy or daddy can't remember how to move certain parts of their body, it is dangerous for them to try to do certain things. They might fall and get hurt. You can be a big help to them by doing what they ask you to do and by not leaving your toys and other things laying around to get in their way. Mommy or daddy is going to need a lot of help while they re-teach their brain what they've forgotten. As long as everyone does their best to help, Mommy or Daddy can focus on getting better. We want Mommy or Daddy to get better, right?

Thank you for understanding and wanting to help. Together we can make Mommy or Daddy all better.

**Actionable Recovery Strategies:**

1. Don't use big words that

require further explanation. But don't talk down to them either.
2. If they are confused and you need to slow down and explain better, you'll likely see it in their eyes. Be an empathetic communicator.
3. To them, this is an adult paying attention to me and inviting me into their world. Eagerly engage with them about your therapy.
4. Before the age of five, no matter how well you explain it, it will likely still be confusing. Answer questions as bluntly and simply as possible.
5. Depending on their age and intellect you may have to repeat this conversation several times

before it sticks.
Repetition, repetition,
repetition.

# Part V: Reach Out [Here's Where You Can Negotiate]

### *Chapter Nineteen: Take a Chance*

By now I may be preaching to the choir. By now you've likely realized that you can't take this journey all alone. You likely recognized that you need help and lots of it. You may not be able to bathe yourself, dress yourself, roll over in bed by yourself, or even shower and use the toilet by yourself. Been there! It's humiliating and decidedly unfair. Still, it may now be your reality. If it is, you own it whether you like it or not. Of course you very probably don't like it. Who would? Even if you were the most-needy person on the planet, you likely wouldn't want to be this needy. Independence is probably very important to you. I get it. You've been robbed. Help, police! Bad things happen to good people. You should find a way to get past that. There's so much more to life than sitting around feeling sorry for yourself. No battle was ever won with self-pity. "So climb aboard and strap yourself in, soldier. It's gonna be a bumpy ride!"

Admitting to yourself that you need help is a good way to start. Recognizing that there is an entire social apparatus out there willing to help is also important. Sometimes it's as simple as just saying, "I'm disabled," and the apparatus starts in motion. Likely, however, you will need to be a bit more assertive than that. You should start with the people around you. I encourage you to be vocal about what you actually need. Do as much as you safely can for yourself, and then let others take up the slack. Be polite, I would be surprised if anyone actually owed you help; regardless of how great you were before the stroke. Help isn't an entitlement for most of us, at least not yet. You'll attract more bees with sugar. You'll attract more flies with crap. Bees are productive and helpful. Flies are just annoying.   Remember you're trying to keep your dignity intact. Being demanding and unpleasant isn't going to do that for you. You should trust that human nature prompts us to help those with a sincere need. Your need could not be more sincere. I encourage you to reach out to those around you and then to church and community organizations. The help available is bountiful. The biggest risk you run is becoming overly dependent on others, and that's a fair trade for what you're dealing with now. You can deal with dependency issues later.

---

## **Actionable Recovery Strategies:**

1. You need help. Don't kid yourself into believing otherwise.
2. Begin with those around you already, your family and close friends. Allow them into your therapy world.
3. Most people want to help someone in your circumstances. Let them in.
4. You must politely petition others for their help. Their help is voluntary and not something you are automatically entitled to.
5. Having taken advantage of your most immediate resources for help, reach out to others in your community, the resources are abundant.

# Chapter Twenty: Friends and Family (you're most immediate source of help)

You know these people love you. They loved you before the stroke and they love you even more now. Lean on them for support. They want you to, they expect you to, and they want to be there for you. You aren't asking them to do anything for you that you wouldn't be willing to do if the roles were reversed. Especially now that you've experienced a stroke for yourself, you would be the first to step up and offer help. Your friends and family are your most invaluable resource. Be careful not to wear them out, however. You know what you can do for yourself and what you can't. As long as you are doing as much for yourself as you possibly can, there's less likelihood of your wearing them out. Just watching you do for yourself will encourage them to want to do more for you. We naturally get a lift emotionally through helping others, so helping you is helping them. Don't deprive them of the benefits of helping you. If you want, you can borrow my personal motto, "I can only do what I can do. I can't do more and I won't do less."

There's an old saying, "If you want to be a friend, do something for someone else. If you want someone to be your friend let them do something for you." You've got everything you need to expand your circle of friends. You have more than enough need to go around. Don't be shy about asking for help. You're probably a great person to be friends with, and helping others provides benefits for the helper and the helpee. You probably have a significant pool of acquaintances just waiting to become friends and the larger your circle of friends the less help each friend and family member needs to provide. Making friends so that you can get help may sound narcissistic, but remember that this is as much for them as it is for you. For reasons I will go into near the end of the book, you will want your circle of friends to be as large as possible.

### **Actionable Recovery Strategies:**

1. Lean heavily on your family and close friends. They expect you to ask for help. If the roles were reversed, wouldn't you help?
2. Be aware of the burden you present and don't overdo it. You will need

these people for a long time. Don't wear them out.
3. Do as much for yourself as safely possible. Seeing you do for yourself will inspire them to help you more.
4. Helping others is a positive experience for the helper. Your recovery will become an investment for them. Let them help you recover. It will be gratifying for them as well.
5. Expand your circle of friends whenever possible.

### Chapter Twenty-One: Church and Community

A simple internet search for "disability help" yields nearly 40 million results. With so many resources out there, you're going to find plenty of help. I personally recommend that you focus some time on the following websites:

**Www.yellowpages.com**
Just enter "disability" as a search term and the name of your city. The site will return dozens of potential resources. The only downside is that many of the results will be insurance companies.

**www.icdri.org/legal/CAP.htm** The Client Assistance Program in your state exists to help you find disability assistance resources in your area.

### **www.abilitylist.org**

Ability List is a site that requires you to contribute, if you want to participate. So be prepared to do a little research in your area for disability assistance. Here you can put your yellow page research to work for you. Resources need not be free to qualify.

### **State disability benefits office**

In the U.S., your state has a department specifically responsible for assisting people in your situation. They probably have an online application, but you may want to call them and fill out the application over the phone instead. Take full advantage of any assistance they can provide to you. Your taxes have been going to pay for this for years. Outside of the U.S., the process is probably similar.

If your church or religious affiliation offers assistance to people with disabilities, your best opportunity for receiving that help is to reach out to them directly. Some religious organizations do not require that you be a member in order to receive assistance. Community and religious assistance programs receive tax breaks, grants, donations and other funding for providing assistance. These programs are there for your benefit, why not accept their generous offer to help you?

Actionable Recovery Strategies:
1. Identify your specific needs and then reach out to one or more of the many agencies and organizations who are ready and willing to help. If your first try isn't a good fit, keep working at

it, you will find the one that's right for you and your unique set of circumstances.
2. The internet is a treasure trove of details on organizations who specialize in assisting the disabled. Don't just accept your circumstances, Google a solution.
3. Start locally, and expand from there. Everywhere you call, ask them who else they would recommend that you reach out to.
4. Government, Non-profit and for-profit organizations, your religious affiliation and many others, have programs directed at addressing the needs of the disabled. Don't just

get help somewhere, get help everywhere.
5. A note regarding Healthcare.gov: if you are receiving disability and that is your only income, you qualify for tremendous discounts on health insurance through the marketplace or your state program. Look them up. (however, keep in mind that if you are collecting disability from Social security then you are required to be enrolled in Medicare and therefore you do not qualify for coverage through healthcare.gov.)

### *Chapter Twenty-Two: Be ready when help is offered*

You will be asked by sincere individuals on regular basis what they can do for you. You may instinctively want to say, "nothing, but this would be a missed opportunity. Always be thinking about what you need help with. If you had a small army of assistants, what would you try to accomplish? You actually do have that small army available to you, but they don't want to butt-in uninvited. They are waiting for you to give them some direction regarding how you want to be helped. You have to take some initiative in this process and be ready with an answer when someone asks what they can do for you. You've heard the saying, "strike while the iron's hot." That is because iron is soft and moldable when it's hot. You can mold this otherwise strong and hard metal into a variety of shapes by striking it while it's hot. The real meaning of the saying is that you need to take advantage of an opportunity when the opportunity is still available.

This will be one of your biggest challenges. You were not likely accustomed to relying on others so much before the stroke. Maybe you took pride in your independence. Your whole world is change now and self-reliance is just another casualty in the mayhem known as stroke. You wouldn't expect an infant to be self-reliant and, since your situation is similar to that of an infant, you shouldn't expect it of yourself either. I know, you're not an infant, you're an adult who has forgotten how to use part of their body. Your point is? Everything about this situation will and should feel wrong. You're playing the game of life, and you've been sent back to the beginning, except that you get to keep the spouse and car full of children. It's not intended to be fair. It just is what it is. Focusing on the unfairness of it all will not solve anything. You have to get past that and focus instead on moving forward. To do that, you're going to need help. Plenty of people in your life are willing to help. You just need to be ready with a list of things you need help with. Be bold and aggressive with your list. Reach for more than just, "can you hand me that cup of water." Try to accomplish something that others can look at as an accomplishment as well.

    Maybe what you need help with is one of your therapies. As a result you will end up with more functionality and, every time you can perform that movement on your own, the person who helped you will recognize it as something they helped you get back. Is it going to change the world? It's going to change your world. Some therapies are not possible on your own. You don't want to miss out on regaining that functionality. Ask for help and accept it when it's offered. Dignity is found in accepting our own limitations and not trying to do more than is reasonable on our own. Admitting you can't do something without help is not undignified. Humility and self-awareness, that's what's dignified.

Actionable Recovery Strategies:
1. You know your needs better than anyone. That means you know how others can help you, even if you can do it yourself. There should never be an

instance where someone offers to help that you don't have a list of things ready.
2. Allowing others to help makes them feel better and it should make you feel more loved and appreciated. We all need that.
3. There is nothing to be gained by dwelling on what you've lost. You will not be rewarded for sitting around complaining.
4. Your dignity is better served by getting up and doing. Especially if you involve others in your efforts.
5. Don't expect more from yourself than you would a toddler learning to walk or eat with a fork. Yes you can do more than an

infant, but you also can't. Accept your reality.

# Part VI: Coping with loss [Acceptance]

## *Chapter Twenty-Three: Career*

You've already realized that stroke is synonymous with change. This may in fact mean you are going to have to let go of the career you have spent a lifetime building. It just adds insult to your injury. You were a competent professional and now you're forced out of your chosen field, not by a more competent professional, but by your own brain. This whole situation could not be more unfair. This is, however, likely not the first time you've had to change careers. You're a resilient human being and you can overcome this setback.

When I lost my job I was already a year into my recovery. My employer decided that I was no longer competent to perform the job that I had done for them for seven years. From my perspective, I still retained all of the knowledge that I had before the stroke. I was not able to type with both hands, but I could still keep up with the workload. The disintegration of my reputation stems from a couple of incidents. First, I had to undergo a surgery related to the stroke that should have been outpatient. It was not. I was admitted to the hospital. I had informed my immediate supervisor, prior to the surgery that I would be unreachable for a few hours that morning and mistakenly assumed that was adequate. Silly me, I had no idea I would be expected to reveal my personal health issues to every manager in the company, and in advance.

    The second incident involved one of the managers of the company not getting a report in as timely a manner as he thought he should, also due to the surgery. The company did not lose any money or experience any public embarrassment as a result of the delay, but the manager insinuated it was a huge problem. Needless to say, I was irritated at the company's decision to let me go; especially given seven years of dedicated service. Ironically, during the termination inquisition, it was suggested that my role was so critical to the company that everyone needed to know where I was at all times. Yet, it wasn't so critical that I couldn't be shown the door. In all fairness, other than this one final act, I had been treated quite well by my former employer and given tremendous opportunities for professional growth. I'll admit to having pursued legal venues, but proving discrimination it turns out, is not as inclusive a process as you might think. I am what a good friend used to refer to as "fish-belly white" and middle aged, and that, it seems, is considered an impediment in discrimination circles. Even if you are disabled.

Ultimately, leaving the office politics behind was one of the best things that could have happened for my recovery. My termination put a lot of pressure on my family financially, and forced my wife to have to go back to work, but the dramatic reduction in stress was a miraculous revelation of what I really needed to get away from. Change is difficult and often messy, but it isn't necessarily a bad thing. Change can be exactly what you need, but because, as human beings, we are resistant to change we fight to keep things the way they are. You may be so busy trying to keep your job that you haven't looked around to see what other options there are. To help you cope with a change in employment or any other change, look at it this way. Assume for a moment that you have lost your job or some other dramatic change has occurred. What will you do now? You'll make the best of a bad situation. You'll make the best career change decisions that you can. Why wait for your career to leave you. If it seems inevitable, bite the bullet and move on. Change can be good and with all of the other change taking place inside and around you, take a "bring it on!" attitude. Embrace change as your new normal.

Actionable Recovery Strategies:
1. Change in your career may just be another aspect of the whole stroke equals change dynamic. Roll with it. I will not quote The Sound of Music, but you know where I'm

headed. Don't resist change. Climb that mountain.
2. Had you embraced change more abundantly before the stroke, it may never have happened. Make friends with change.
3. Change has always been your companion. You can cope with any change that comes your way. Those with the most dignity, never complain about or resist change.
4. Look change squarely in the eye and say, "bring it on!"
5. If recovery is a journey, then change is the landscape that unfolds before you. Treat change like something to be curious about. Figure it out.

## *Chapter Twenty-Four: Yourself*

You may only be aware that you have changed because of observations others have made. Changed you are, nonetheless. It may be slight or it may be dramatic. Regardless those changes have set you on a new course and affected your relationships. Doubtless you're looking askance at any change in yourself, but for the same reasons that change in employment can be a good thing, change in you can be good too. Again, it can be messy and there may be collateral damage, but when you learn to embrace change you start to find the good in it and not put up as much of a fight.

Before my stroke I was a very type "A" person. I thrived on stress and intentionally went looking for it. I was determined to have everything my way and bring everyone around to my way of thinking. I worried about everything. Fast forward nearly three years and my wife still accuses me of not caring about anything. I am laid back to an extraordinary level. Far from seeking out stress, I avoid it whenever possible. The biggest stress in my life now is wondering if people will buy my book. I remember that other stressed out guy, and you can't pay me to go back to who I was. The stress aspect of my pre-stroke life seems like a nightmare to me now. Even now, as I look back on who I was, I tense up. Despite my continued disabilities and the various challenges that have come from the stroke, in some ways I am more content with my life now than I ever was before. Are there still things I would change? Absolutely, but for the most part my quality of life is better.

I could list off any number of things that are wrong with my life, as it stands, and the list would be longer than my arm, my good arm. I'm sure that you could generate a similar list for your own life. Focusing on that list will not bring either of us any happiness. Everyone can point to aspects of their life that could be better. In that respect you're completely normal. The key to maintaining your dignity is in focusing instead on the changes that are good, and oh, there are good changes. Once you take a step on the journey toward gratitude, you suddenly see all kinds of good that you never noticed before. It's remarkable how many good things happen in everyone's life on a daily basis. As you start to recognize these positive influences in your own life they will begin to multiply before your eyes. It is a funny fact of life that focusing on gratitude, makes us more aware of things to be grateful for. A new you can definitely be a good thing.

Actionable Recovery Strategies:
1. Embrace change in you and everything around you. Change happens regardless of what you want or do. Change can be a very good thing.
2. A new you could be better for you and everyone around you, but the new you may not be in the mold you created for yourself in your pre-stroke life. Embrace the change.
3. Stop adding to your list of things in your life that are wrong. There is no happiness there.

4. Look for changes, and find the good in each one. You'll be surprised how it improves your mood.
5. If you are naturally a negative person, that was never a dignified aspect of your personality. Time to change.

### *Chapter Twenty-Five: Friends and Family*

Your personal change may have impacted what you used to have in common with others. If your relationship with someone is based on a shared interest, the stroke may have taken that interest away from you. Now things may be awkward and uncomfortable between you and this person. Rather than struggle to maintain the relationship without a common interest, it may be time to re-evaluate the relationship entirely. I'm not suggesting that you simply tell the person to get lost. Instead you should be open with them regarding the change you've experienced and how it has affected your enthusiasm for the previous commonly held interest. Let them know that you still value their friendship a lot and that you want to explore what other common interests you may share with them now. Who could possibly be offended by that? On the other hand, pretending to still be interested in something you're not, will most certainly strain your relationship with that person.

Maybe that person is your spouse, and maybe that common interest used to be sex. Now you're compounding the complexity of the problem to extraordinary proportions. As human adults, especially men, we tend to tie a great deal of our personal worth to our sexuality. You've probably heard this but a disproportionately large number of strokes lead to divorce. You aren't the same person you used to be and that is going to place a huge strain on your relationship. Perhaps the nerve damage you have experienced has re-wired your sex drive. If you're a woman, you might be able to pretend it isn't a problem. If you're a man, not so much. To further complicate the issue, sex is as much emotional as it is physical. Just because the old tingly sensation isn't there anymore, doesn't mean that the emotional need for sex has gone away. You may in fact be putting a lot of effort into jump starting your sex life, but no amount of medication or stimulation seems to help. That can really suck.

    Remember, however, that change is good. Take this opportunity to work on aspects of your relationship that have been overshadowed or neglected, due to sex. There is so much more to a full and rewarding relationship that doesn't involve physical contact. Trust me, I know how difficult it can be to say goodbye to sex.

Maybe it isn't even about you. Maybe the changes you've undergone have affected the way your spouse sees you sexually. Try taking sex off of the table. Good things come to those who wait, I believe that. Talk about it, mutually agree that you're going to take a vacation from sex for a while. Give yourselves a chance to become reacquainted. The new you is as complex as the old you was. Don't unravel an entire marriage over something as trivial as an orgasm. I assume you didn't marry a prostitute, don't expect your spouse to act like one by having sex with someone he or she feels no attraction to. You're not less of a person for not having sex regularly and neither is your spouse. Step back and see the bigger picture. No one ever died from a lack of sex, however many people have died from too much of it. Value your relationship on the basis of loyalty and compassion, not on an instinctual drive. The emotions and passion associated with sex can be explored without engaging in anything that leads to an orgasm. Give yourself more credit than that. You're not an animal, you're a rational, thinking human being. You can reason your way through this. Be grateful for and celebrate the non-physical aspects of your relationship. Gain a greater appreciation for your spouse on a whole new level.

I can greatly appreciate that this is easier said than done. Your brain tells you that you already have a relationship that includes physical intimacy, but your brain's been wrong before. If you want something to trust, trust all of the signals you're getting. Change often happens in a big way here. So, how do you start from scratch re-building a marriage? There are volumes of books dedicated to this subject and I won't pretend to have all of the answers. I will instead share my own experience. Early in our relationship my wife and I had a big blow up. In the aftermath of that argument we both agreed that we would eventually forgive each other for what the other might have done. We decided that since forgiveness was inevitable, we would extend it in the moment and not wait. This has been the cause of a tremendous amount of harmony over the years. I encourage you to let go of resentment and embrace the change. It may be the best thing that ever happened to your relationship.


Actionable Recovery Strategies:
1. Relationships will change. Be

open with the other person. Don't try to hide your change, that never works out.
2. A change in your sex life is not necessarily a bad thing. Use it as a motive to explore other aspects of your relationship.
3. Relationships are an ever evolving dynamic (change). You should accept that, if you have changed, and you have, then your relationships have changed as well.
4. Your commitment to your relationships will carry you through any rough patches.
5. Rely on your higher power to help you navigate any choppy waters.

## Part VII: Be Inspirational
## [Getting Past the Grief]

### Chapter Twenty-Six: Without Even Trying. You are an Inspiration.

It's not hard to inspire, we are inspired every day by numerous sources. We see an ad for a hamburger and we immediately want one. We drive past a sign announcing 2 for $1 candy bars and we stop in to buy our favorite. I have intentionally not looked up the definition of inspire, but this is what it means to me.

*Inspire means to motivate someone to think, say or do something they were otherwise disinclined to do.*

You may not think that it's your job to inspire others, but inspiring is part of your reality now. Every day that you stick around and continue to push through this trial, you are an inspiration to others; and that's just by being you. Why not embrace this new role and turn it into a mission or purpose in life? Imagine how rewarding your life will be if you spend all day every day trying to inspire others. That's not the same as trying to impress others. Your inspirational ability comes from your quiet perseverance. Making your best effort to improve every day. You don't have to lift a car over your head or solve world hunger. You just need to be the best you possible.

    You haven't even started, and you're already doing it. How hard could it be? Being your most diligent, most dedicated, most hard working self will inspire others to not give up on the challenges that they face. What you have to overcome looks monumental to those who haven't experienced it. It may seem monumental to you as well, but you've already seen the improvement that comes from even a modicum of effort. You have every reason to be optimistic about the future. Your enthusiasm and perseverance will be infectious to those around you. You are a one person movement toward a better world. Too many people say to themselves, "I'm just one person. What difference can I make?" If 800,000 additional people every year make it their daily goal to inspire others to keep moving and never give up, imagine the positive change that could be accomplished. You're not just one person. You are a part of everyone around you. Be the best part. Be the inspiration.

Actionable Recovery Strategies:

1. Just by being you, you inspire those around you. Thanks to the stroke, you are an inspiration. Capitalize on that, and be the best you possible.
2. Inspiring others will not take a lot more effort. You just need to be dedicated to doing what you can.
3. Maybe you never wanted to be an inspiration, but the stroke has changed that. Roll with the change. Trying to hide from the inspiration that you are, will not give you back your dignity.
4. You are a part of everyone around you. Be the best part you can be.
5. Be an inspiration.

### Chapter Twenty-Seven: Just a Little Bit More (A little extra makes all the difference)

Even if you are by your very nature a negative and depressed individual, your potential for inspirational effect is tremendous. If you, who never see the good in anything keeps pushing forward under difficult circumstances, those around you cannot help but be inspired to give a little more to overcoming their own challenges. I'm not suggesting that you change your personality. If you suddenly became bubbly and energetic, your friends and family might assume that you have had a psychotic break. Then you wouldn't be inspirational. You'd truly be a freak show. No, you need to be you. Just bump it up a notch. Force your stroke to become the source of inspiration that everyone around you needs. Take this monumental pile of crap that you've been handed and spread it around to encourage others to grow. You can do this. It just takes a little more effort on your part.

You're about to turn a corner and the view from there is much nicer. Just a little bit further. Now turn. There, now you see that this stroke isn't your punishment, it's your opportunity. How will you be remembered? This is the moment when you decide. What you chose to do from this moment forward will define how others see and remember you, how you see yourself, and how much dignity you can lay claim to. The path ahead will not be easy, but it will be tremendously rewarding. Your improvement potential will get a boost, your outlook on life and your situation will improve. People will respond more positively toward you and will want to help and be part of the miracle you've come to represent. This isn't just a moment of decision, this is a moment of truth. If you're convinced, cap it off by telling yourself, "I can do this. I can try a little harder and turn my tragedy into a fountain of inspiration for myself and the people I care most about."

    That's the hard part, making the commitment. Actually doing the work will be self-reinforcing. The harder you try, the more persistent you are, the greater the results you'll start seeing. Not just in yourself, but in everyone around you. Seeing those results will just inspire you to try that much harder. Yes, I'm saying that you are becoming your own inspiration. Who could have imagined that when you started to read this book, that by the end you will have become your own source of inspiration and become part of an effort to effect positive change in the world. There's still a long road ahead and the path won't be easy, but you can do this. You are already an inspiration, just keep it up and give it a little more gas. The world needs you and the inspiration you naturally bring with the struggles you face. Show the world that it takes more than a few lost brain cells to keep you down. Rise above this pile of crap and be the inspiration that we both know you can be.

Actionable Recovery Strategies:
1. Everyone has challenges they need or want to overcome. Your example will give them courage to try harder.
2. Life has handed you a pile of crap. Spread it around by being an inspiration

and everyone around you will grow.
3. Dignity is not something you project. It is your right to claim it by your everyday choices. Tell yourself, "I choose to be dignified. I choose to be an inspiration.
4. The effort to be an inspiration is self-reinforcing. The harder you try to recover, the more you will recover and the more others will grow.
5. Rise above the crap. Everyone needs inspiration, especially you.

### *Chapter Twenty-Eight: But I'm Tired*

Of course you're tired. That's part of the whole problem. But your tiredness doesn't come from exertion, it comes from your brain's attempt to compensate for the damage that has been done. That doesn't make the tiredness less real, but it should help you to understand that trying harder isn't going to make you more tired. It may, in-fact, help you to rest better. If you've been internalizing our discussion so far then your whole perspective on recovery may have changed. Moving forward you'll have more reasons to celebrate and more energy to invest in your recovery. If you need to, breathe a great sigh of relief. You have a mission and a purpose that makes everything you've been through and are going through worth it. This stroke, with all of its challenges is a gift. Don't be selfish with it. Share it with the world in the way you persistently and inspirationally deal with it. You may always feel tired, but when it comes time to rest, will you rest with ease? Tiredness is your body's way of telling you that it isn't inspired. Laugh in the face of your tiredness. Tell it to look at you, look at everything you've already accomplished and be amazed at what you're about to accomplish. Inspiration? You are inspiration. Say to your tiredness, "Stand aside and watch what I can do."

    I understand tiredness. Left un-checked, my body generally will try to sleep twelve to fourteen hours a day. I need to take stimulants to stay awake the rest of the day. When I am awake, I spend the majority of my time writing and doing coursework for the PhD program I'm enrolled in. If you're struggling through the day to stay awake, I totally empathize. But what I've found, in my own struggle, is that no amount of tiredness can hope to match the source of inspiration you are becoming. Tiredness, schmiredness. Go out and inspire yourself. Give yourself a reason to get out of bed. You have got people to inspire, you don't have time for tiredness. You've been given this time to change the world's perspective of you. You've been given time to change hearts and minds. You are an inspiration whether or not you want to be. Be the best inspiration you can manage. Show the world what is possible, if you just put forth the extra effort. There are so many reasons in this world for people to be pessimistic. There is a serious deficit of inspiration. Your timing could not be better. Hurray, you've managed to become inspirational just when the world needs it the most. Imagine the awesome changes that are about to take place all around you. Tiredness should be the least of your worries. You're on a quest now and there's no time to waste. Pack your bags, the adventure s just beginning. There's a whole world out there that needs your inspiration right now. Go inspire others by just being you. Look at you, you've already inspired me to write this book. Thank you!

Actionable Recovery Strategies:
1. Tiredness is just a fact of stroke recovery, but its only perception. You don't need the amount of rest you're getting. Push through the tiredness. Find reasons to be awake.

2. Sleep is a great way to escape the unpleasantness of life. However, it is also a great way to escape responsibility. Don't abuse sleep.
3. Don't condition your brain to think that sleep is the best way to cope with anything unpleasant. It will come back to bite you.
4. What you need are reasons to stay awake.
5. Find the inspiration you need to push aside your tiredness.

**Part VIII: More with Less [Rebuilding Your Life]**

### *Chapter Twenty-Nine: Embrace Life*

You've been through a lot, but you're still here. That means you're not done. There is more for you to do. Embrace that fact. Love it! Any day you wake up should be a good day, because you're in it. With the rising of each new day comes new hope and an opportunity for great things to happen in your life. Your attitude, and the perspective through which you view the world around you, will shape the experiences you have. No one but you can decide what kind of a day you're going to have. You are the writer, director and star of this movie. You are the captain of this ship. Pick a course and stick to it. Intentionally plot the destination for your day and move toward it. Every journey of a thousand miles begins with one step or one rotation of the wheels on your chair. Obstacles are your opportunity to inspire and reclaim your dignity. You have been given a gift. True, it's wrapped in a lot of unpleasantness, but it is a priceless gift nonetheless. Cherish the opportunity before you. If you ever got a new bicycle for your birthday, could you have imagined, on that day, all of the adventures that bike would carry you to in the following months and years? No, a stroke isn't exactly a shiny new bike, but it will carry you to many amazing adventures that you otherwise wouldn't have had and introduce you to amazing people you would have never otherwise met.

    Maybe you're inclined to view your stroke as a burden and an inconvenience. That is your prerogative, it's your stroke and you can make of it whatever you want. They are your lemons. You can pucker up and swallow the juice straight, or you can add sugar and water to make some refreshing lemonade. It's entirely up to you. Choosing to see the good in this tragedy doesn't cost you anything except your cynicism. The rewards, however, are tremendously greater for choosing to be optimistic. When the movie of your life reaches its final scene will it close a glorious epic journey, or will it be the last of a long string of disappointments. This is the moment for you to decide what the remainder of your life will stand for? What meaning will you assign to your stroke? Will it be a catalyst for awesome, inspiring achievements or does it herald the beginning of a tragic end. Sitting around, waiting to die is easy and requires no effort on your part. I hope that you'll choose to be inspirational. It can and you'll have to work at it every day, but you can do hard things. You know it and God or the universe know it. That's why you're still here. Make the most of this opportunity. I promise, you'll be better off for having done so.

Actionable Recovery Strategies:
1. Any day that you wake up is a good day. Find the reason to be present in that day. You have work to do.
2. Obstacles are opportunities to reclaim your dignity.
3. The direction your life takes today is entirely your choice. You can't choose the obstacles you'll face, but you alone can decide how you'll respond to them.
4. You can inspire yourself, and you can inspire

others, but only if you choose to push forward.
5. See your stroke for what it is, an opportunity to inspire.

## *Chapter Thirty: Deny Discouragement*

I believe that courage is a decision to press forward despite obvious challenges, as well as unknown hurdles. Dis-courage is, in my view, the tendency to give up. Moving forward, you will likely exist in a place somewhere between the two. Discouragement will pull at you and try to draw you over to its side. Courage will beckon to you, but won't try to force or drag you over to its side. It's easy to allow yourself to be dragged into discouragement, just don't do anything. You have to make a conscious choice to be courageous. It requires action on your part, which makes courage a verb. So courage moves, while discouragement sits idle and does nothing. Yes, watching T.V. and playing electronic games all day is doing nothing. Reading, except for social media, is better because it expands your mind, but it's still an idle escape. To truly be courageous you need to engage in the world. Connect with people face to face. Get to know them on a personal level. Share the intimate details of your recovery with them. A courageous person opens up to others. Don't over share, there are limits to what people need to know about you, but the more they get to know you the more opportunity you will have to inspire them.

    Feelings of discouragement will always surface. It's a natural response to exercising courage. Whether or not you experience discouragement isn't important because you will experience it regardless. The key to continued courage is in not giving in to the discouragement when it comes. Treat it like what it is, life pushing back. Just say, "Okay that didn't have the desired effect, so I'll try something else." Or even better, "I don't care if life didn't like that. I'm doing it anyway!" Remember Sir Isaac Newton's third law of motion states, "for every action, there is an equal and opposite reaction." Discouragement is, therefore, a natural response to courage. If your attempts at courage lead to discouragement then you applied courage correctly. SUCCESS! Just like multiplication and division can be used to check each other, you can use discouragement as a tool for verifying your correct use of courage. That may seem a little confusing, so let me put it this way. If you try (courage), and you fail, you will likely feel discouraged, which only means that you tried correctly and Newton's third law is manifesting itself. Keep trying. Variations of this saying abound, but the original source is disputed, regardless it applies perfectly to both of us. "You only truly fail when you fail to truly try."

Actionable Recovery Strategies:
1. Courage is a choice, discourage is the absence of choice.
2. Choosing courage won't isolate you from discouragement. Choose courage every time and you leave no room for discouragement to take hold.
3. Every choice you make will trigger some form of opposition.
4. Don't let discouragement take hold. It isn't your friend.
5. Only when you don't try, do you truly fail.

## *Chapter Thirty-One: Silver Linings*

It is said that, "every grey cloud has a silver lining." I suppose that means that you can find good in bad circumstances. You've probably met someone who is always looking on the bright side of things. Annoying, I know. I have observed that for them it's a defense mechanism, it's how they cope with disappointment and push away discouragement. They insist on dragging the rest of us into their process. I'm not suggesting you become that person. No one needs to know what's going on in your head when you refuse to allow disappointment to lead to discouragement. However, when you're alone or with someone you trust, you should vocalize whatever affirmation kept discouragement at bay. Your brain needs to hear you say it. Silver linings aren't a refusal to accept reality, far from it. Silver linings are selecting the reality you wish/desire to live. Isn't that self-delusion? It depends. If you lie to yourself to avoid the pain of reality then yes, you are delusional. However, if you simply chose to find the real good in a real bad situation then you are choosing a different reality. Ignoring the bad in favor of the good is delusional. Ignoring the good is equally delusional. Seeing both the bad and the good and choosing to emphasize the good is healthy and will inspire you and those around you to greater things.

    The real question here is why do gray clouds have a silver and not a gold lining? I suppose it's because silver is gray. Gray clouds equal silver. Does it really matter? It's figurative, which means you won't actually find either metal in a cloud. That explains why clouds don't routinely come crashing down. Which is also why you don't hear this conversation very often.

Question - "What do you see in that cloud?"
Answer - "Death!"

Silver linings are synonymous with perspective, which is how you view the world. Does the world change because of the way you see it. Absolutely! You are as responsible for the world around you as everyone else, and one person with a positive attitude can shift the mood of everyone around them. So when you choose to focus on silver linings you are actually choosing to change the world into a more positive place, which spawns more silver linings. Looking for and finding silver linings results in more silver linings for you to find, and soon your world is a much better place for you and everyone around you.

Actionable Recovery Strategies:
1. Speak out loud the affirmations you focus on to push away discouragement. Your brain needs to hear you say them.
2. No situation is totally bad. Look for the positive in any circumstance you find yourself in. You'll like the "you" that results.
3. Mine the clouds in your life for the positive they have to offer. As you look for good, you'll find it more often.
4. You can change your perspective of the world simply by choosing to look for the good. The world

around you won't change, but you will change the way you see it.
5. By focusing on the positive, you inspire yourself and others to see the good in the world.

### Chapter Thirty-Two: Surround Yourself (You can never have enough friends)

Misery loves company—so the saying goes—and we all know what birds of a feather do. While you're in the mode of recreating your world in a new and more optimistic way, you may want to consider the company you keep. Do your companions share your quest for silver linings or are they focused on the gray cloud and expecting it to come crashing down on top of them at any moment? As you recreate your world you'll want to surround yourself with like-minded people. Not to suggest that you should be closed minded or non-inclusive. Rather I believe that you can accomplish very little if you're focused on silver linings while everyone around you is focused on the clouds. You either need to change your crowd or covert them. This is where being inspirational comes in handy. Even if this new silver lining mentality is a stark departure from your more traditional pessimism, you can inspire others to share your perspective. Share with them what you're trying to do for yourself and for them. Don't be annoying about it, but give them the benefit of your epiphany.

    Suddenly a courageous choice becomes a movement. That's when your world begins to improve dramatically. Why did I write this book? I've been where you are. I know how tough it can be. No, my experience is not exactly the same as yours, but it's been close enough for me to feel your pain, your discouragement and your loss. I want you to know that you're not alone and this isn't the beginning of the end. This the beginning of the rest. This chapter of your life has not been written for you. Like any heroic character, you've been given a setting and a list of challenges to overcome. We are all watching anxiously to see how you'll handle it. The drama of life doesn't come from the obstacles we face, but from the way we chose to face them.

Actionable Recovery Strategies:
1. Catalog the attributes of those people who lift your spirits when they're around. Then practice emulating those attributes, so that you can lift yourself when they aren't around.
2. Share with those around you, how you are trying to improve your perspective. Be informative about it, not annoying.

3. Help those around you to see the silver linings. Improvements in their perspective will come back to you and help your perspective.
4. You and you alone can decide how you will face your challenges. Decide once and for always that you want to see the positive in every circumstance.
5. Turn drama on its ear by choosing to see the silver linings. Drama is not a fact of life, it is simply another perspective. Choose differently.

## *Chapter Thirty-Three: Freak of Nature*

I've intentionally saved this bit of truth for last. For the vast majority of human history people with disabilities were tucked away where they were neither seen nor heard. That's assuming they were even permitted to live. The disabled were a socially unacceptable subset of society. They weren't expected to contribute anything and so they were permitted to consume very little. They were considered to have no hope for any quality of life, so there was no reason to cater to their needs. Frankly, with all of the resources available to us now, the attitude of the general public has not really changed all that much. We're no longer tucked away, but most people go out of their way to not see us. We still aren't expected to contribute and many people resent us for what we consume.

That is the dark truth about the world we live in. The expectation that we don't contribute often yields to the great lie that we are incapable of contributing. Even those who acknowledge our ability to contribute often convolute the fact with something like, "Well, to the extent they're capable." As if that isn't true of every human being. No one can contribute more than they are capable.

It has been my experience that when someone experiences a deficiency in one area that they compensate in other areas. Otherwise where did the phrase, "getting by on good looks," come from. Your disability has likely lead to an increased ability in other aspects of your life, and in those aspects you have an increased ability to contribute. Adversity is a natural result of living. When you made the choice to live, it's as if you thumbed your nose at nature, who in turn responded, "Oh yeah, well we'll just see about that." Choosing to live an inspirational, courageous and dignified life runs contrary to what nature expects you to do. History consigns you to the shadows and nature expects you to stay there.

You, however, are a freak of nature. You won't be content to stay in your little corner. You will be a force to be reckoned with. Nature and the rest of humanity will have to deal with you. You have a lot to offer. In some respects your disability has made you supernatural. You won't contribute less than a person without a disability, you'll contribute as much, if not more. Stand back world, here you come.

Prepare to be amazed and inspired, world. Your contribution will be awesome. Your disabilities don't define you. You're in charge and you decide who you are and what you can do.

Thank you, again. You're the reason I chose to write this book. You're are my inspiration! In my view, you have tons of dignity and infinite potential. You're going to beat this and in the process inspire the world around you. Don't give in to discouragement or fatigue. Look at what you've already accomplished. You can do hard things. You've got this!

Actionable Recovery Strategies:
1. It should not shock and upset you when someone acts toward you with contempt or a lack of empathy. As a species we have more growth to

accomplish in that area. However, you can be the inspiration for that growth.
2. Like all human beings, you can only do what you can do, but don't let others define what you're capable of. Step out of the shadows and re-define what the word disabled means for those who expect less.
3. Don't use the narrow minded perspective of others as an excuse not to try. You may be deficient in some areas, but you've likely compensated in others. Show the world what you're capable of.
4. The stroke has turned you into a supernatural individual. Like all super heroes, you have

weaknesses and you have strengths. Let those strengths shine and inspire.
5. You can do hard things. Go out and conquer your challenges. You can do it!

www.ingramcontent.com/pod-product-compliance
Lightning Source LLC
Chambersburg PA
CBHW060829220526
45466CB00003B/1028

# CLASSIC SUDOKU

## BOOK 3

**www.goldpuzzles.com**

Published in 2020 by Gold Puzzles

© Copyright 2020 Gold Puzzles

All rights reserved. No part of this publication may be copied, photocopied, reproduced, or translated, in whole or in part, without the prior written consent of the publisher.

The contents of this publication are believed correct at the time of printing. Nevertheless, the publisher can accept no responsibility for errors or omissions, changes in the detail given or for any expense or loss thereby caused.

If you would like to comment on any aspect of this book, please contact us at contact@goldpuzzles.com.

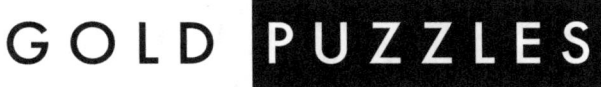

# Get your **FREE** print-at-home puzzle book at

## subscribe.goldpuzzles.com

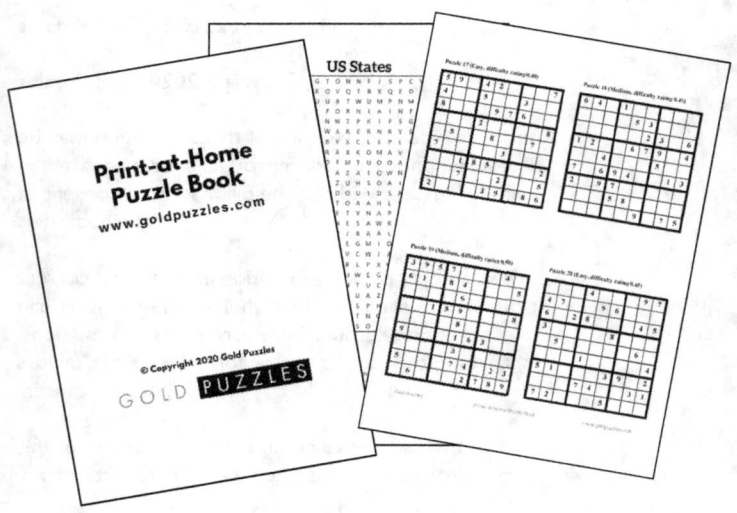

www.goldpuzzles.com